This journal belongs to

_____

THE
CHRISTIAN
MOM'S
Pregnancy
Journal

Week-by-Week Guide, Prayers & Memory Book

AUBRY G. SMITH,
CD & CBE (CBI)

ZEITGEIST · NEW YORK

Published in the United States by Zeitgeist, an imprint of Zeitgeist™,
a division of Penguin Random House LLC, New York.
penguinrandomhouse.com

Zeitgeist™ is a trademark of Penguin Random House LLC

ISBN: 9780593435502

Illustrations © Natdzho/Creative Market, ussr/Shutterstock.com,
and Olga_Angelloz/Shutterstock.com
Interior design by Brooke Johnson
Cover design by Aimee Fleck
Author photo by Joseph Taub
Edited by Lauren Ladoceour

Printed in the United States of America

1 3 5 7 9 10 8 6 4 2

First Edition

CONTENTS

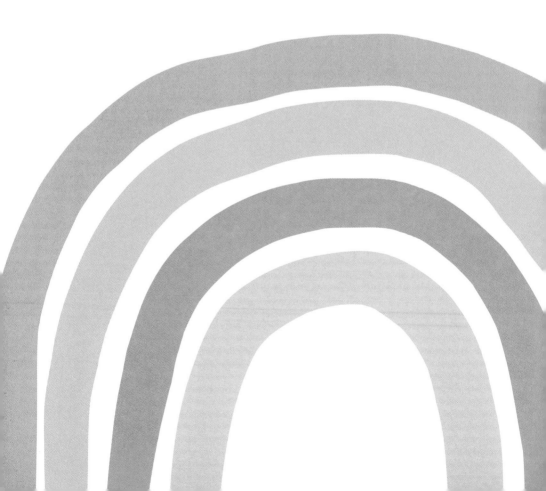

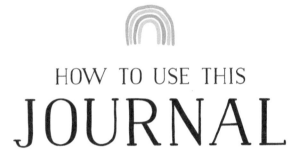

HOW TO USE THIS
JOURNAL

Congratulations on your pregnancy! Whether this is your first or eighth child, a wild surprise or meticulously planned, pregnancy is a profound season that deserves to be celebrated and recorded. This journal is designed to help you process the many emotions and milestones of childbearing before God. In it, you can track your experiences, feelings, thoughts, and prayers as you bring new life into this world.

Throughout the Bible, visual reminders were vital to the people of God. Rainbows in Genesis, river stones in the book of Joshua, Passover celebrations, and the sacrament of the Lord's Supper all served as remembrances of God's acts. These memorials allowed believers to reflect on God's faithfulness in the past, which gave them hope for the future. This journal, commemorating your journey with God through pregnancy, can work in much the same way.

As a childbirth educator, birth doula, mother, and theologian, I have seen how God uses pregnancy for deep spiritual transformation in the lives of women and in my own life. God gives us the opportunity to learn to trust Him throughout the ups and downs as well as experience sublime joy in Him. As parents, we learn anew the depths of the Father's love for us as His children. Pregnancy is the start of the sacrificial love for our children that mirrors Christ's self-giving love for us. Journaling and studying Scripture through your pregnancy are ways of bringing yourself and your experiences before the Lord so that He can transform you.

In this journal, you'll find 40 weeks of Biblical reflections on pregnancy, childbirth, and motherhood. Each week contains a short introduction that explains where you and your baby are in your journey, both physically and spiritually. You'll also find a passage from the Bible, a prayer, and a journaling prompt for you to meditate on as well as space for you to record your thoughts and prayers. Along the way, you can also paste in pregnancy photos, ultrasound pictures, or other keepsakes from your pregnancy.

The journal begins in week 5 of pregnancy, assumes 40 weeks of gestation, and takes you through the early postpartum weeks. However, the "standard" timetable may not be your baby's timetable! Should you find out you're pregnant after week 5, feel free to go back and play catch-up or simply begin right where you are. So, too, you may have your baby before week 40—or perhaps a bit after. Likewise, the weeks following your baby's birth can be a bleary-eyed blur, and journaling may be the last thing on your mind. Be gentle with yourself. The goal is to be transformed in Christ, not to finish an assignment!

My prayer for you is that through pregnancy, birth, postpartum, and motherhood, you will experience God's presence in the sacred work of creating and nurturing new life. There is no perfect pregnancy and no perfect mother, but you follow a perfect God who promises He will be with you through every step of the road ahead.

IN CASE OF UNEXPECTED LOSS

Sadly, some women experience miscarriage in their pregnancies. For others, grief comes by way of a still-birth. If this happens, I am so sorry. Even though you have never gotten to know your little one, the loss you experience is as heavy as any other. Find ways of memorializing your baby's brief life, such as giving them a name and making a keepsake—perhaps saving a page from this journal that encourages you. While you may not understand why the Lord has allowed this to happen, be sure to pour out your heart to both Him and a trusted loved one to help you get through.

PASTE
ULTRASOUND
HERE

FIRST ULTRASOUND

YOUR GROWING
MIRACLE

Welcome to your first trimester! Your mind may need time to catch up to the reality of your pregnancy. Perhaps you don't even look very pregnant this trimester—at most, you may appear as if you've had a large lunch! For many women, the first trimester can be tough as their bodies respond with a dramatic flair to the new little person growing inside. These next few weeks of journaling and devotions will help you process before the Lord the many changes going on in your body, your mind, and your soul. They may also help you begin to comprehend that this is, indeed, happening. Rejoice!

WEEK

5

Your baby might be as tiny as a sunflower seed this week, but they are making themselves known! Many newly pregnant moms experience telltale signs that it's time to take a pregnancy test: exhaustion, swollen breasts, and nausea. For your baby, this is a critical time as their heart and neural tube—what will later become the brain and spinal cord—are forming. In addition to nurturing your baby, God also wants to nurture your heart during this special season. When you come to Him as you truly are—without a mask of any kind—He can grow you into greater maturity in Christ.

Children are a heritage from the Lord, offspring
a reward from him. Like arrows in the hands
of a warrior are children born in one's youth.
Blessed is the man whose quiver is full of them.

Psalm 127:3–5a

A HERITAGE FROM THE LORD

In these first weeks of pregnancy, it's normal to experience a bombardment of conflicting emotions. You may be both thrilled and terrified, joyful and overwhelmed. Whatever your circumstances, one of the most important things you can do is to bring all of yourself, and your baby within you, to the Lord. With Him, you can find peace for your churning emotions and joyful strength for the road ahead.

Throughout Scripture, God clearly cherishes children. They are not a nuisance, a drain on resources, or a commodity to collect. Children are a gift we receive from a generous and good God. Perhaps you wholeheartedly receive this goodness, as this is a child you longed for. But maybe you don't *feel* the goodness and blessing yet. Or maybe you're somewhere in between. That's okay! You can ask God to grow your faith as you walk with Him in His truth.

Psalm 127 begins, "Unless the Lord builds the house, the builders labor in vain." God is building your house; He is intimately involved in your life, your family, and your womb. God's provident work in opening and closing wombs is a major story line throughout the Bible. The fact that you are pregnant is not a mere result of natural processes; your pregnancy is *from the Lord*. Pregnancy is not a mistake or a coincidence, nor is it something we can control or make happen all on our own.

God's view of parenting is also different from the world's perspective. We all want to leave a legacy, but a heritage from the Lord carries eternal weight. God is giving you, through your child, an arrow for your quiver. As followers of Jesus, our purpose is living for His glory, not our own. As a mother, you have been given a profound task in raising this child you now carry. Your little "arrow" needs to be lovingly cared for and shaped so that they may be shot out as a powerful instrument of God's love in this world. But you do not bear the burden on your own. The Holy Spirit, who lives within you, will empower you to be the mother your child needs you to be. God's goodness is ahead; receive it!

A LITTLE PRAYER FOR YOU

Lord, give me faith in Your goodness on this journey.
I cast all my cares and emotions on You, receiving
Your peace and Your love for both me and this
child. Holy Spirit, grant me wisdom and impart
upon me the eternal purposes of mothering.

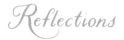

Reflections

How did you discover you were pregnant,
and how did the news make you feel?

Your baby is about a quarter of an inch long now and looks like a little tadpole. Their heart has begun beating, but you may not be able to hear it on a Doppler just yet. You may be researching your health-care provider options this week. Pray for God's direction, as the team you choose can make all the difference in your prenatal care. Your health-care provider can also help you navigate your new nutritional guidelines, but don't stress if you can't keep much down these days. God designed your body to nourish and protect your little one through morning—and sometimes noon and night!—sickness.

Adam named his wife Eve, because she would become the mother of all the living . . . and she became pregnant and gave birth to Cain. She said, "With the help of the Lord I have brought forth a man." Genesis 3:20, 4:1

PARTICIPATING IN CREATION

As the "mother of all the living," Eve held a unique role in God's creation. In Genesis, God made every living creature on earth merely through His speech. Humans, however, were different. He made Adam from dust, then took a rib from a sleeping Adam and formed Eve from the rib. When Eve birthed her first son, she marveled at this miracle: with God's help, Eve herself had actively participated in creation. She was given the honor of co-creator, mirroring God's own creative power to bring life to the third human.

You are also participating in creation with God as Eve did! God is in the process of creating an entirely new life, and you are the one He has chosen as His co-laborer. Did you know that God has given you the remarkable role of displaying the image of the Creator in your very body? According to Genesis, all humans are made in the image of God, which means that in various ways, we reflect who God is. We think, we show emotion, we are relational. God gave humans dominion over the earth as extensions of His own benevolent care. But God grants women the privilege of participating in His creation in a very special way. He works with your body to form life inside you.

From the outside, it may not seem as if much is happening, and you may not have even made your pregnancy public knowledge yet. Inwardly, however, your body is working with God in the secret places to form a new creation. The whole process brings glory to our Creator—your pregnancy is an act of worship, as you do exactly what God has created your body to do.

As your body experiences changes, so, too, will God transform your heart and soul through pregnancy, childbirth, and mothering. God is shaping *you* into a new creation as you live your life before Him. Pregnancy is beautiful, but it isn't always glamorous. Nausea, bloating, gas, and other symptoms can cause you to focus on the bothersome aspects of this season and to potentially miss the beauty of what God is doing. Take some time this week to appreciate the hard work your body is doing with God to make a whole new person and to marvel at the privilege of being a co-creator alongside Him.

A LITTLE PRAYER FOR YOU

God, thank You for choosing me as Your beloved co-creator. I give all of myself over to You—body, mind, and soul—to be transformed into the image of Christ. Please safely direct the formation of my baby's heart and neural tube this week.

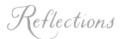

Reflections

How do you feel about God creating through you, and in what ways can you worship Him for His goodness and His creativity?

_____

_____

_____

_____

_____

_____

_____

_____

_____

_____

_____

_____

_____

_____

_____

_____

_____

_____

WEEK 7

This week, your baby's umbilical cord is forming to connect to your body in a new way. They'll soon receive nutrients and oxygen through this cord from the developing placenta. Your little one hasn't grown much in length from last week, but your baby now has webbed hands and feet, and God is developing their brain more intensively. Speaking of brains, yours might feel foggy, tired, and forgetful as "mom brain" sets in. Bring your and your baby's mind before the Lord this week, asking Him to renew yours in His truth and to guide your baby's into healthy development.

"Come to me, all you who are weary and burdened, and I will give you rest. Take my yoke upon you and learn from me, for I am gentle and humble in heart, and you will find rest for your souls." Matthew 11:28–29

RESTING IN JESUS

Pregnancy can be exhausting! Your body is engaged in intense work with God, creating and nourishing the tiny life inside you. You may find that even a nap each day (if you can get one!) and going to bed early each night still leave you dragging through your normal tasks. If you have children underfoot, health ailments, and/or a demanding work schedule, the weariness can feel unbearable. Your energy will return in the second trimester, but what about *right now*?

Jesus cares deeply about those who feel weary and burdened, whatever the cause. He doesn't call them to pull themselves up by their bootstraps, grab some coffee, and quit whining. He doesn't say, "Try harder!" and shake His finger at them in disappointment. He gently beckons them to simply come to Him to receive the rest that only He can give—a rest more effective than naps and caffeine could ever be.

The image of taking on Jesus' yoke is familiar to the original audience but likely more foreign to us. Imagine a pair of oxen yoked together to plow a field or cart a heavy load. Together, they share the work side by side, easing the other's burden. Jesus offers the weary and burdened the opportunity to take off their own oppressive, exhausting, and lonely loads and join Him. His yoke brings rest deep into our souls, where we need it most. His rest frees us from striving to be perfect, put together, and peppy. We can come to Him just as we are.

Jesus also calls His followers to learn from Him when they take on His yoke. What can we learn from His gentleness and humility of heart? Can we learn gentleness for our own selves in this tiring season, rather than pushing ourselves to be as productive as we usually are? Can we learn the humility that comes from dependence on the Lord and others when we find ourselves at the end of our own resources?

Consider your current burdens, your worries, and your own physical exhaustion. Perhaps you can list them out in the journal space provided. Close your eyes and listen to Jesus say to you through Scripture, "Come to Me and find rest." Offer up your list of burdens and ask Him to give you His yoke and His rest, deep down in your soul.

A LITTLE PRAYER FOR YOU

Lord Jesus, thank You for being my Good Shepherd, caring for me and giving me the rest I truly need. Thank You for carrying my burdens alongside me. Break through my brain fog so that I can meditate on Your truths and guide the development of my baby's brain this week.

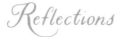

Reflections

What burdens can you give to Jesus to receive His rest?

Your baby is about a half inch long now and growing at an incredible rate. God is forming their eyes, nose, and sweet little cheeks to look more baby-like. Your baby has begun to make tiny movements, but it will be a while yet before you can feel them. You might be feeling more bloated this week, you may be craving or detesting certain foods, and your moods might be unpredictable. Be gentle with yourself and ask the Lord for His help with how you treat others. Remember that we don't need to hide our anger, sadness, or frustration from Him—He already sees it all!

Do nothing out of selfish ambition or vain conceit. Rather, in humility value others above yourselves, not looking to your own interests but each of you to the interests of the others.

Philippians 2:3–4

FINDING HUMILITY IN MOOD SWINGS

Your hormones are all over the place, and you may be experiencing intense mood swings as a result. The smallest offense may set you off into a frenzy of rage or a flood of tears, and the lack of control over your emotional responses may frustrate both you and the people who love you.

The good news is that God can use mood swings to grow you into deeper spiritual maturity. Pregnancy is an extremely formative season—both physically and spiritually. We often wear masks before God and others, concealing our true selves, but pregnancy hormones may disintegrate these masks! Imagine mood swings as an opportunity to bring all your anger, sadness, confusion, and frustration before the Lord. Ask Him to help you make sense of these feelings and to help you respond in a godly way with self-control.

In this week's verse, Paul's words to the Philippian church call all believers to imitate Jesus Christ as they relate to one another. It takes great humility to look beyond ourselves and to truly care for others more than our own interests. Paul goes on in this chapter to describe Jesus' rights to all glory—but that He gave them up in love, giving His own life on our behalf.

Pregnancy is intense discipleship time. You are growing a new person, and you are experiencing the surrender of your own interests—and your very body—for the sake of someone else. Be careful not to let a sense of martyrdom and entitlement grow in you. Yes, your body is working hard, and you need extra care in this season. It can then be tempting to expect everyone around to serve and attend to every new need, and when those needs aren't met, disappointment sets in.

Rather than giving your heart to martyrdom, ask God to help you as you relate to both your baby and those around you with sacrificial love, just like Jesus. Consider how you might serve those around you in humility, rather than expecting to be served.

Finally, if you find that your emotions are too overwhelming, consider reaching out to a friend, a pastor, or a counselor. We were never designed to walk alone. Sharing your burdens and mood swings may make them much easier to bear and may help others give you grace.

A LITTLE PRAYER FOR YOU

Prince of Peace, I ask that You give me Your peace,
even in my moodiness. Help my mindset be as
Christ Jesus, caring for others in true humility. Use
this pregnancy to help me get rid of my masks
that hide my true self from You and others.

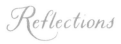

Reflections

How has this pregnancy affected your emotions? Record your funny (and maybe not-so-funny) reactions to your wild hormones in the space below.

WEEK

9

This is an exciting week, since the heartbeat of most babies can now be heard on a Doppler! This thrilling experience makes the pregnancy seem more real. Your baby is about a whole inch long now, but your jeans may protest that the baby is much bigger as your uterus has grown up out of your pelvis. Many women grieve the loss of the ability to button their pants. They know it's a good thing, but our culture so idolizes thinness that it can be a tough adjustment. This week's devotional can help orient your heart around offering your body up for the Lord's use.

"I am the Lord's servant," Mary answered. "May your word to me be fulfilled." Luke 1:38

SWEET SURRENDER

What an emotional moment when you get your first glimpse of those pink lines on a pregnancy test! While you may be filled with excitement, your mind may also race with the many changes ahead of you and a loss of your sense of control. Your body begins expanding, often in places you wish it wouldn't. You may crave strange foods at an intensity that demands to be satiated. You may have irrepressible nausea that affects your daily routines. Pregnancy, childbirth, and motherhood can be profound reminders of what was true all along: we are entirely dependent upon God, who alone is sovereign and in control.

Jesus' mother, Mary, displays a beautiful example of giving over her body for God's service. As a young, unwed girl in the ancient Near East, she knew pregnancy outside of marriage would have been detrimental—if not fatal—for her. In a culture where honor was everything, women were in danger of being stoned to death for bringing shame on their families, and Mary's entire family's honor was at risk in their small community. Yet God was asking Mary to entrust all of that to Him in order for her to bear the Savior of the world. Mary's response in the preceding verse is one of profound trust and submission of her entire being to God.

You probably don't face the same dangers in your pregnancy that Mary did, but it's likely that God is asking you to give up control in some areas of your life and to entrust those things to

Him. Perhaps your finances are on shaky ground and bringing a child into this situation seems impossible. Those without a partner have to consider the practical side of solo parenting. Maybe you worry about your maternal skills, your time, your job, or your future.

What are those parts of your heart that you may be grasping tightly to maintain control? Can you release them to God in faith, trusting that He is truly on His throne both over the universe and over the details of your life? The discipline of submission to God is a powerful antidote to our natural instinct to control and manipulate. It's a discipline that brings freedom to us as we place ourselves under the loving care of our sovereign Creator.

A LITTLE PRAYER FOR YOU

God, would You show me the places in my life where
I am clinging to control rather than entrusting
everything to You? Give me strength to release my
grip on what I cling to, so that my hands may be
free to cling to You in full, trusting submission.

Dear Baby

Write a letter addressed to your child about what it means
for you to trust God and to be His servant.

Your baby is about one and a half inches long this week, and their bones are beginning to take shape and give their body structure. Their teeny stomach is even producing digestive fluids! Have you given much thought to your hopes and plans for labor and childbirth? It may seem like a long while away, but it isn't too early to begin praying about the birth. Where you will give birth, who will be with you, and even how you want to give birth are things to research and plan now. Remember, in Jesus, you have the blessing of God upon you as you go through pregnancy, labor, and birth.

The Lord gives strength to his people; the Lord blesses his people with peace. Psalm 29:11

PEACE IN PREGNANCY

Through the very process of childbearing, God has enacted His program for redemption. In Genesis, because Adam and Eve ate of the tree of the knowledge of good and evil, sin broke their intimacy with God and marred His good creation. Consequences were delivered, too, and to this day, some teach that the challenges of pregnancy and childbirth are nothing more than a reminder of God's punishment for original sin.

The fuller truth, however, is that God also promised that a Savior would come through Eve and that Eve's offspring would one day crush the head of the serpent. Centuries later, Jesus, the ultimate blessing, came to earth and bore the condemnation that our sins deserve. God's wrath against sin was not poured out on us but on Jesus on the cross.

So remember, through Jesus, you have access to God's peace, comfort, and life—even as you labor. You are not cursed but loved to the greatest depths. As it says in the book of John, God loves you so much that He gave His own Son to bring you life. And He lovingly allows you to bring life as well.

In Jesus, the kingdom of God has come but not fully. Theologians call this "already–not yet," where we have a blending of both the effects of the Fall and the glory of God's wholeness. Yes, there may be pain and a difficult struggle in labor, but it is not a curse or the wrath of God poured out on you. It may be the baby's position or your body's signals that you should move around or a sign that you need medical attention. No matter what your future birth feels like, God will be with you to bless you, not to hurt you. As this week's verse says, He has promised to give you strength and bless you with peace.

How you view childbirth—and God, who designed it—may affect your experience of it. It may surprise you to know that many women have had beautiful, peaceful, and fearless births in which they felt the presence and pleasure of God. Begin praying this week for God to show you His blessing throughout your pregnancy and as you start to mentally prepare for labor. Remember that He created you and created your body to be able to deliver your child. He can give you strength to bring your child into the world.

A LITTLE PRAYER FOR YOU

Father God, I know that You give Your people strength and peace for whatever they face, including childbirth. Give me wisdom as I begin thinking about my birth plan, and help me know that You are for me in childbirth, not against me.

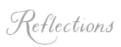

Reflections

What kinds of questions or fears do you have about birth right now, and how can God's peace and blessing meet you in those fears?

_____

_____

_____

_____

_____

_____

_____

_____

_____

_____

_____

_____

_____

_____

_____

_____

_____

_____

_____

_____

_____

WEEK
11

Your baby is about two inches long now, and the little webs between the fingers and toes are disappearing. Their face is becoming more their own—ears, nose, and mouth are all shaping up and in the right places now. Your little one is beginning to form a unique set of fingerprints on those miniature fingers, and it's astonishing to think about God's one-of-a-kind design for not only your baby's body but also their life. Pray this week for your baby as God creates their features and also, by His grace, the good works in which your child will walk.

For we are God's handiwork, created in Christ Jesus to do good works, which God prepared in advance for us to do. Ephesians 2:10

CREATED FOR GOOD WORKS

In his letter to the Ephesians, Paul clearly lays out the basics of the gospel: because of God's great love and mercy, while we were dead in our sins, He gave us life through Christ. Paul is careful not to attribute our salvation to good works—salvation comes only by grace, through faith, as a gift from God. No one earns gifts; they are given freely. But God "created [us] in Christ Jesus to do good works" in response to His extravagant grace. Our good works reflect our good God and bring Him glory as we become the people He created us to be.

The holy work of motherhood is a million opportunities to walk in these good works, prepared for us by God. You will serve a small person in humble but necessary tasks—diaper changing, feeding, cleaning up, correcting. You will sacrifice sleep, comfort, and perhaps a certain dress size for the interests of another person. You will learn deeper ways of loving someone else and giving yourself for their good. You will bring your child up in your faith, teaching them about a God who loves them and showing them what it looks like in your daily life to be faithful to God. The good works God prepares for us in advance certainly include these selfless, giving works that you do for your child.

It is marvelous to think about the tiny person inside of you, a unique individual never before created, whom God is putting on this earth for a purpose. What are the good works that God is preparing for this child? Of course, we can't know or predict what the Lord will do in this child's life, but one of the most powerful things you can do as a parent is to pray for your child. Pray for their childhood years, that they will develop a relationship with God early on and learn to trust Him. Pray for their teen years, that independence from their parents will lead to greater dependence on the Lord. Pray that they would fulfill the Lord's calling to bring glory to Him in all that they do. And pray that God would enable you to be a parent who always points your child to Jesus. You won't be a perfect parent, but you can point your child to the One who gives grace abundantly.

A LITTLE PRAYER FOR YOU

Lord God, Your handiwork is incredible, and I praise You because both my baby and I are created to reflect Your goodness. I ask that You empower me in the good works You've laid out for me, so I can be an example to my baby as they learn to follow You.

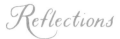

Reflections

What are some of the good works that you know God has prepared for you to do?

_____

_____

_____

_____

_____

_____

_____

_____

_____

_____

_____

_____

_____

_____

_____

_____

_____

_____

WEEK
12

A little over two inches long now, your baby looks like a tiny human rather than a tadpole! Your baby has grown some fuzzy hair all over their body and is beginning to make sucking movements with their mouth. Many women begin to feel some relief from their early pregnancy symptoms around this time, and if they haven't already, they're also contemplating how to tell their friends, family, and employer their big news. Ask the Lord for wisdom this week in sharing your pregnancy, especially with those for whom it might bring up pain of a desired but yet unreceived child.

Who can proclaim the mighty acts of the Lord or fully declare his praise? Psalm 106:2

SHARING YOUR GOOD NEWS

The fog of the first trimester is lifting, and your bump may be getting more difficult to conceal—if you wanted to hide it! Many women wait until the end of the first trimester to inform others of their coming baby, and if you are one of them, you may be bursting to tell your good news to the world. You may be considering how to reveal your pregnancy in your own unique way. Many women think of clever "I'm expecting!" announcement photos to post on social media as a way of bringing others into their joy and excitement. Others plan a special party or gifts for the siblings, grandparents, aunts, and uncles in the baby's life. If you prefer to keep it simple, that's okay too!

Proclaiming to others what God has done is an important part of the Christian life, and you can consider the miracle of your pregnancy as part of that calling. God's miraculous work may be easier to see if your pregnancy was preceded by difficulty conceiving, but it is certainly no less true for any other pregnancy. The conception and the formation of your child are truly a miracle, and they are the "mighty acts of the Lord" that we should proclaim! Let your praise of His incredible work in your life and in your womb always be on your lips.

For some who hear your pregnancy announcement, your news may land with sharp bitterness in their hearts. Why has God granted this child to you but not to them? This should not diminish your joy, but you can ask God for compassion and grace for these hard conversations. How can you encourage others to see the mighty acts of the Lord in their own lives and to declare His praise, even as they grieve the things He has not yet done?

Soon, it will be obvious even to strangers that you're expecting, and your pregnancy will be the thing that everyone wants to talk to you about. Consider how you can direct conversations to giving praise to the Lord in this season of your life. What is He teaching you as you co-create with Him? How are you experiencing God in new ways as you bring both your excitement and your fears to Him? Our whole lives are meant to be lived in worship to the One who made us—pregnancy is no different.

A LITTLE PRAYER FOR YOU

Jesus, open my mouth to declare Your praises with joy and thanksgiving. Thank you for this baby and for the work You are doing in me. Please grant me compassion and wisdom as I share with those who do not receive my news with joy.

Dear Baby

In the journal space, write a letter to your baby detailing
how you shared the news of their arrival with the world.
How did people react?

Congratulations! You've made it to the end of the first trimester! Your baby's vocal cords are now formed, ready to soon fill your ears with coos and screeches. At three inches long, they are growing at a rate of about a half inch per week. Your head may be spinning with the number of decisions ahead of you: Hire a doula for the birth? Get an epidural or not? Breast milk or formula? Stay home or continue working? Take courage from the knowledge that the Lord is with you and that He loves to give wisdom to His children.

"The Lord himself goes before you and will be with you; he will never leave you nor forsake you. Do not be afraid; do not be discouraged."

Deuteronomy 31:8

OUR GUIDE IN THE STORM

Pregnancy and parenthood can be filled with uncertainty. *What if I face complications further along? What if I'm not strong enough for childbirth? What if I can't provide for this child? What if my baby isn't healthy? What if I'm not a good parent? What if I don't know what I'm doing?*

While both joy and pain are on the road ahead, the Bible can help you find a straight path through rocky terrain. The reality is that life contains hardship and uncertainty; however, Scripture tells countless stories of people who faced true adversity to guide us in our own lives. Some people put their faith in God, while others chose to rely on other things—and found them to be unworthy objects of trust. Trusting God with your own life can be challenging enough; trusting God with your child's life may be even more difficult.

Our natural instinct is to flee from discomforts—perhaps by bingeing a TV series, endlessly scrolling social media, or mindlessly eating. Like a fly buzzing around your ears, however, anything you may be trying to avoid will continue to pester you until you look at it and deal with it. But when you face the things that worry you and measure them against what God says in His Word, you may find that they shrink before His greatness. He goes before you in all things and remains with you throughout your life.

Pregnancy will change the way you think about the world in drastic ways. As your mindset changes, it's important to continue training your mind in the truth of God's Word. You can allow your anxieties to overtake you, or you can fix your hope and trust in Jesus, your anchor in all storms. When trials come, you may not automatically turn to Jesus. You must train in the off-season, so to speak. In what ways are you preparing your heart to hold firmly to Christ should any of your fears be realized? Are you developing your prayer life, memorizing Scripture, finding fellowship and mentorship from other mothers? How are you anchoring yourself *now* in the truth of God's presence in all circumstances?

Remember that between the joy and deep love that are ahead, there will also be hard work. No matter what arises, God's presence is what will give you the courage to meet it all head-on, and He will guide you through the storm.

A LITTLE PRAYER FOR YOU

Father God, I lay all my fears at Your feet. You are worthy of my trust and my hope as I consider my future with this baby. Give me confidence, knowing that You go before me in life and in parenting.

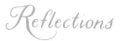

Reflections

What fears or uncertainties about the future
do you need to bring to the Lord today?

NAME IDEAS FROM THE BIBLE

Scripture says, "A good name is better than fine perfume" (Ecclesiastes 7:1a). Names carried great significance in Biblical times. In several instances, we see God changing someone's name as He changes the course of their life. When He made a covenant with Abram's family, God changed Abram's name ("exalted father") to Abraham ("father of many nations"). In other instances, names tell us something important about how God relates to a person. Hannah means "grace," and in answer to her prayers, God surely showed her grace in granting her a son. Jesus' name means "God saves," and God's plan to save humankind permeated Jesus' life.

Choosing your child's name can be a decision that invests deep meaning into your child's life. Their name can reflect what you hope and pray for their character, their future, and their relationship with God. The Bible is full of names brimming with deep significance—here's a list to get you started!

ELIJAH—"My God is Yahweh"

ISAAC—"He laughs/rejoices"

JOSIAH—"Yahweh supports"

JUDAH—"Praise"

MICAH—"Who is like Yahweh?"

EDEN—"Delight"

HOSANNA—"Save us"

MERCY—"Compassion and forgiveness"

SHILOH—"Tranquil"

ZION—"The mountain where Jerusalem is," also used to mean "heaven"

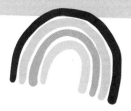

PASTE
PHOTO
HERE

BUMP PHOTO

PASTE
ULTRASOUND
HERE

ANATOMICAL ULTRASOUND

MARVELOUS CHANGES

Praise God for the second trimester! For most women, this trimester is the most enjoyable as their energy increases and the nausea fades. Excitement builds as you feel those first kicks and tumbles, possibly find out the sex of your baby, and grow a rounding belly that brings a smile to strangers. Joy and gratitude come most easily in these weeks, and it may be easier to get back to your normal spiritual routines, such as attending church, doing more thoughtful Bible study, and focusing your prayers. The spiritual work you do now will reap a harvest in your and your baby's life later!

WEEK
14

Your baby is about four inches long now. In addition to the "peach fuzz" (lanugo) all over their body, they are likely beginning to sprout hairs on their head. The external genitalia are developing so that by next week, a skilled ultrasound tech can tell you what you're having—unless you want to be surprised! As for you, if your exhaustion and brain fog have finally lifted, you may be able to engage in new worshipful wonder. Offer up your praise to God as you consider His delicate and intimate work in knitting your child together, as He once knit you together.

For you created my inmost being; you knit me together in my mother's womb. I praise you because I am fearfully and wonderfully made; your works are wonderful, I know that full well. My frame was not hidden from you when I was made in the secret place. Psalm 139:13–15

KNITTED TOGETHER

In our world of factory-made goods, we can richly appreciate the intimacy and care involved in hand-knitting something together. In knitting, the creator holds their project close as they weave the yarn in and out, over and under. Through the painstaking and meticulous labor of the designer, something new takes shape. The knitter chooses this particular color here, that pattern there, and lovingly creates a beautiful new piece of art.

This artistic "knitting together" is the imagery David chose to describe God's creation of his own body within his mother's womb. Psalm 139 is a wondrous portrayal of God's intimate nearness in every aspect of David's life—his sitting, rising, speaking, and thinking. God oversees every element of development, even in the darkness of the womb. Biology is full of sacred processes designed by God, and the creation of a baby within their mother is one of the most complex and magnificent of these.

Many of us tend to think of God as far-off and inaccessible. But this is not what the Bible reveals to us. Our God draws near to His people. He rescued the Hebrews from slavery, then set up the law and temple as a means of bringing them back into His presence. He sent food and water to the Israelites when they were desperate and calling out for help. He even sent His Son, also knitted together in a woman's womb just as we are, for the reconciliation of God with humanity. Our God has come near to us, and He's always right there with you.

God is also very near to your baby in your pregnancy. He is knitting—not manufacturing—your baby's ears, fingers, and toes into His own design of artistry that could never be replicated. He is taking care over His creation, considering, loving, and nurturing your baby.

Have you ever felt like God is far-off? Maybe you're even feeling that way right now. Challenge yourself to take some time this week to read and meditate on Psalm 139. What passages strike your heart most intensely? Why? Consider writing those verses on an index card and keeping it with you (and memorizing it!) as a reminder of God's nearness and His loving care for you and your baby. You might even keep it visible during labor to remind you that just as you didn't create this baby alone, so, also, you will not labor alone.

A LITTLE PRAYER FOR YOU

Lord, thank You for Your creative artistry in designing and knitting together my baby in my womb and even my own body in my mother's womb. Thank You for Your nearness to me in every phase of life. When I feel alone, open my eyes to see where You are.

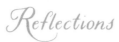

Reflections

What moments of God's nearness to you in this pregnancy
can you write down as a reminder when He feels far-off?

_____

_____

_____

_____

_____

_____

_____

_____

_____

_____

_____

_____

_____

_____

_____

_____

_____

_____

Your little one is measuring about four and a half inches this week. They are busy working new muscles to kick, twitch, suck, and swallow, though you may not be able to feel any movements quite yet. Many women find out their baby's sex this week, and some even plan a gender-reveal party to invite their friends and family into their joy. Some women, and perhaps even you, may display a preference for one or another, especially if you have other children. Receive this new child as they are—a gift from your knowing Father.

Every good and perfect gift is from above, coming down from the Father of the heavenly lights, who does not change like shifting shadows. James 1:17

THE BIG REVEAL

Prior to the relatively new technology of ultrasound, many cultures developed their own methods of discovering a baby's sex, such as through special ceremonies or rituals, by analyzing what the mother ate, or by studying how the mother carried the baby. All these methods had about a 50 percent chance of accuracy! In Scripture, sometimes parents found out what they were having through an angelic announcement. Abraham, Rebekah, Samson's parents, John the Baptist's father (Zechariah), and, of course, Mary all had this experience. But for most women throughout history, their baby's sex remained a mystery until just after birth.

What an incredible time in history and technology that you can learn the sex of your baby before birth with such a high degree of accuracy! Many people, maybe even you, feel that waiting to find out at birth is a thrilling and suspenseful experience. They often buy gender-neutral clothing and accessories that will also work for any siblings that may come later, which is convenient and budget-friendly. For others, learning the baby's sex can help them prepare if they want to decorate the nursery a certain way. Many women treasure the experience of buying sweet ruffled dresses or tiny boots and bow ties while pregnant. Knowing might also help you narrow down a name, and calling your baby by their name as you talk to them can give you a greater sense of bonding.

Some women experience a twinge of disappointment at the gender reveal—perhaps one they might never admit to anyone else. Or maybe you have family members or friends who are outspoken about which you "should" have—as if you could decide! As you bring these things to the Lord, you can ask Him to help you and your loved ones receive this child as a gift from a loving and knowing Father. He can help melt away your disappointment into joy and gratitude for your baby.

Whether you decide to learn your child's sex during your pregnancy or right after birth, seeing your growing baby on an ultrasound is a remarkable moment. You may be able to catch them sucking their thumb or toe, playing with the umbilical cord, or sleeping in a certain position that they favor even after birth. Be sure to save an ultrasound photo in this book as a reminder!

A LITTLE PRAYER FOR YOU

Father, please give me wisdom about whether to
find out my baby's sex now and how to share that
knowledge with others. Thank You for the gift You
are giving me in this child. Continue to develop their
little body with Your loving and attentive care.

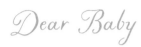

Dear Baby

If you're discovering the sex of your baby during pregnancy, write a letter to your baby about that moment. If not, share with your child why you decided not to!

Your baby is about five inches long now, and your little "bump" is really beginning to show! Your baby might be sucking their thumb, a habit that will strengthen their mouth muscles for feedings outside the womb. Can you feel fluttery little kicks yet? In this week's devotional, we'll look at the powerful prayers of a mother for her child. Perhaps you might use the tiny kicks you're beginning to feel as a reminder to pray for your baby. Pray for yourself, also, that you would have faith to entrust your child to the Lord.

"I prayed for this child, and the Lord has granted me what I asked of him. So now I give him to the Lord. For his whole life he will be given over to the Lord." 1 Samuel 1:27–28

PRAYERFUL PARENTING

Hannah is one of the many women in the Bible who received children from God after a period of intense, unfulfilled longing. Her story, found in the first two chapters of 1 Samuel, is one of trustful waiting and hopeful prayer. Perhaps the child you are carrying is the result of years of waiting and prayers. Maybe you are battling negative feelings toward a pregnancy you didn't feel ready for, or you are worried about the years ahead of caring for a child. No matter the situation, the best response is to imitate Hannah. Her empty arms drove her to cast herself upon God with such fervency and desperation that the priest Eli thought she was drunk! All her hope was centered on God, and she maintained faith in His generosity to her.

When Hannah received the answer to her prayers in the birth of her son Samuel, she committed another act of deep trust in the Lord: she gave her son up to the Lord's service just after he was weaned (likely around age three or four). In giving over her young son, she released to the Lord any control or claim she had over Samuel's life. Hannah's faith-filled entrusting of her son to God provides a powerful example to us mothers today.

Follow in Hannah's footsteps by praying for your child, starting now and continuing throughout their life, surrendering your baby to God's loving care. Who else will pray for your child as much as you will, and who else loves your child as much as God does? If you let Him, God can grow you into a spiritually mature woman as He makes you a mother. In each moment of excitement and each moment that seems beyond you, the Lord waits for you to entrust your child to Him—the only One who can truly give this child what they need.

We can't always keep our children safe and protected. But we can follow Hannah's example of entrusting our future and our children to the Lord through fervent and sincere prayer. Pray for their health, their spiritual growth, their future friends, and their future spouse. Pray for the Lord to speak to them and to guide them in His ways. Your prayers for your child may be the most significant thing you do as their mother.

A LITTLE PRAYER FOR YOU

Holy God, You alone have granted me this child, and I pray for the faith to offer them back to You. I entrust this child to You, for Your service. Empower me by Your Spirit to be a mother who is deeply rooted in prayer.

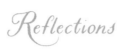

Reflections

In the space below, write out your prayers for your child and offer your child up to the Lord in an act of trust over their future.

Your baby's ears are developing quickly this week, and now they can hear you! Babies establish a strong bond to the sound of their mother's voice, so feel free to talk, sing, or even read stories to your little one. As you become more visibly pregnant, you may notice that strangers suddenly feel more connected to you and want to help you. They may also feel free to give unsolicited advice or even touch your belly! It's difficult to know how to respond to such attentions, but the Lord can help you balance maintaining appropriate boundaries and enjoying the extra attention and connection your baby brings with others.

Therefore, as God's chosen people, holy and dearly loved, clothe yourselves with compassion, kindness, humility, gentleness and patience. Bear with each other and forgive one another if any of you has a grievance against someone. Forgive as the Lord forgave you. Colossians 3:12–13

COMPASSIONATE CONNECTIONS

As your body reveals to the world that you're carrying new life, you'll notice that people are rushing to open doors for you, offering to carry heavy things for you, making small talk with you, or just smiling at you. Many women marvel at how *nice* the world suddenly seems. People often feel an instant connection to those who are pregnant or who have babies, and this phenomenon can be a wonderful reminder of the blessing and joy of a baby.

Sadly, not all the attention you receive will be positive. People might share their unsolicited opinions on what your body should look like or whether you should have an unmedicated birth or an epidural. One woman I know was chastised by a pharmacy tech because she had a pineapple in her grocery cart, which the tech felt that pregnant women should never eat! Unfortunately, these comments often carry into parenthood: You're holding the baby both too much and not enough. You're enabling your toddler's tantrums, and you're also not letting them express their emotions. You're simultaneously giving your teenager too much freedom and sheltering them. With such confusing advice, it's difficult not to grow frustrated.

Thankfully, Paul's instructions to the church in Colossae can help you navigate this new connection with others. When you "clothe [yourself] with compassion, kindness, humility, gentleness, and patience," you take a step back from your defensiveness and frustration and see the person in front of you with new eyes. Many people make comments as a way of connecting with you and saying, "I've been there! There's so much to know! Let me help you!" Most likely, these people just want you to have a healthy pregnancy and succeed in parenting.

If you're feeling criticized, the buildup of many such comments can harden your heart toward those who might be genuinely reaching out. You may also be particularly sensitive to perceived criticism when it comes to your body, your pregnancy, or how you parent. Paul encourages believers to bear with one another and to forgive as they've been forgiven by God. As you receive advice and opinions, silently ask the Lord to give you His eyes for that person and to grow you in compassion, kindness, humility, gentleness, and patience. Ask for His help to forgive and for the humility to listen when appropriate. But treasure those positive comments and connections with new people—they are a kindness from the Lord!

A LITTLE PRAYER FOR YOU

Lord Jesus, thank You for the new kindnesses among strangers. I ask You to clothe me in compassion, kindness, humility, gentleness, and patience for what feels like criticism. In my own strength, I can let my frustrations get the better of me, and I need Your help.

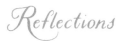

Reflections

Record some of the comments or advice—both helpful
and crazy—you've received during this pregnancy.
Are there people you need to forgive or bear with?

Your baby is about five and a half inches long now and is beginning to form sleeping patterns. Their nervous system is also developing furiously this week, expanding their ability to explore the world with their senses (though their world is quite limited right now!). Many women experience low blood pressure midway through pregnancy, so you may be feeling dizzy at times. Be sure to stay hydrated, check in with your health-care provider regularly, and report any concerning symptoms. Now is also a time to find encouragement and camaraderie in talking to other mothers who can point you to Jesus in this season.

Walk with the wise and become wise, for a companion of fools suffers harm. Proverbs 13:20

FINDING MOTHER-MENTORS

Many women have grown up with incredible examples of motherhood surrounding them—their mothers, grandmothers, aunts, neighbors, and friends from church. But for others, the familial landscape may seem more desolate, full of examples of what *not* to do in parenting. In either case, it's important to find other mothers you respect to befriend and learn from. It's a treasure to find women who have shown with their lives and advice how to be a good mother.

Scripture again and again demonstrates the value of "walking with the wise." Joshua shadowed Moses for many years, learning how to become Israel's next leader. The prophet Elisha learned from Elijah's itinerant ministry. Jesus chose 12 men to follow Him and learn from Him, and the apostle Paul wrote many instructive letters to his protégés in churches around the Mediterranean, continuing what he began with them in person. These wise leaders poured their knowledge into the next generation, recognizing that nobody gains wisdom in a vacuum.

In the book of Titus, Paul urges the older, more experienced women to teach the younger women to love their husbands and children by being an example in their own lives. These are the women who are so important to spend time with as you consider the kind of mother you are growing into. How do these women pray for their children? What are some ways that they teach their children about God and how to live as a Christian? What do they wish they would have known, or done differently, when they were where you are now? These relationships don't need to be formal question-and-answer sessions, though. Watching these women in real life dealing with toddler tantrums in public, negotiating through school drama or technology with older children, or interacting with their teens can reveal important lessons for you. Walking with the wise—living life with them, praying with them through their own struggles, and observing their relationships—is how we ourselves become wise.

You might protest that there are no such women in your life right now. Pray for the Lord to provide them and to open your eyes to those who might already be there. There may be a wise mother to learn from in an unlikely place. Wise people never became wise on their own. We need examples to watch and learn from in every season but especially in parenting, when we need so much wisdom.

A LITTLE PRAYER FOR YOU

Father, please place wise women in my life who can walk with me through life's complications and confusions. Help me to humbly receive advice from others, with discernment in the wisdom You provide. Give me open eyes to see examples of godly mothering around me to learn from.

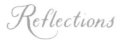

Reflections

What have you learned from other women as you've
watched them mother their children?

_____

_____

_____

_____

_____

_____

_____

_____

_____

_____

_____

_____

_____

_____

_____

_____

_____

_____

_____

Your baby is clocking in at six inches long this week, and a protective waxy coating called vernix caseosa is beginning to form on their skin. Vernix regulates body temperature and helps protect your baby from constant exposure to amniotic fluid. Most likely, it will be present on your baby at birth. As your belly grows, you may experience ligament pain in your lower abdomen. Maintaining a regular exercise routine that includes gentle stretching can help ease this discomfort. If regular exercise and eating well do not come easily to you, ask the Lord for His help. He loves your body and wants to help you care for it!

Do you not know that your bodies are temples of the Holy Spirit, who is in you, whom you have received from God? You are not your own; you were bought at a price. Therefore honor God with your bodies. 1 Corinthians 6:19–20

HONORING GOD WITH YOUR BODY

Pregnancy often gives you a new appreciation for your body. It's marvelous to look in the mirror and see the beautiful, rounding bump that signifies new life. Before, you might have wanted to hide your stomach, but now you're celebrating it and buying clothes that accentuate it! Your skin might have a new glow, your hair might be more luscious, and your breasts might be fuller. Your body's strength and creative power—how it can grow and nourish a new little person—are amazing. Maybe for the first time in a long time, it's easier for you to see your body's beauty.

Pregnancy can also cause feelings of frustration with your body. Pregnancy slows you down, prevents you from easily tying your shoes, and gives you heartburn and sleepless, uncomfortable nights. Innocent acts, like pointing your toes, can lead to painful leg cramps, and the strain on your back may feel like you've aged 10 years in just a few short months. It seems like you're constantly fighting against your body or that it's fighting against you!

Remember, however, that bodies are not bad or evil but created by God as good. They are to be cared for with honor rather than physically (or verbally!) abused. God came to us in the physical body of Jesus Christ—a real body that grew and needed to eat and sleep. The Holy Spirit dwells in our bodies, not just our hearts and minds, and as such, our bodies act as sites of God's presence on earth as the temple once did. Bodies are important in our faith. And although you may be enduring discomfort now, one day God Himself will resurrect our bodies and infuse them with a new glory, and we will be with Him forever.

Instead of dwelling on the new pains that pregnancy is causing, let your pregnancy remind you of the holy work God does in bodies. Your body is now the sacred site of God's creation, and that's quite profound. Is it hard for you to appreciate and honor your body as God's good creation? What are some things you can do for your body that honor it as a site of God's presence and work? Take some time this week to thank God for what He is doing in your body and ask for His help in taking good care of it.

A LITTLE PRAYER FOR YOU

Lord, I thank You for creating this good body that
You've given me. Help me care for it and honor it
as something You bought with the body of Your
Son. I pray for my baby's body that You would grow
it into a healthy body that will honor You.

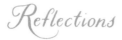

Reflections

Reflect on the changes your body has undergone so far.
How do you feel about those changes, and what
can you do to care for your body?

_____

_____

_____

_____

_____

_____

_____

_____

_____

_____

_____

_____

_____

_____

_____

_____

_____

_____

_____

_____

_____

For many women, this week marks the halfway point of their pregnancy! Your baby is measuring about six and a half inches from crown to rump, and many health-care providers schedule a major ultrasound this week to check babies' development. What a thrill to see your baby's body in detail and to see their little mannerisms. Your baby is most likely starting to work on their sucking reflex, and you might even be able to see them suck their thumb! This scan also detects developmental concerns or disabilities. Bring all your joys and fears before the Lord; He will walk with you through whatever comes.

He tends his flock like a shepherd: He gathers the lambs in his arms and carries them close to his heart; he gently leads those that have young.

Isaiah 40:11

HE CARRIES YOU

Motherhood has always been challenging, but the instant access to vast amounts of information we have today magnifies the challenges rather than reduces them. With the rise of social media, the judgment and shame associated with potentially making a wrong choice can be paralyzing. Mothers want to do what is best for their children, but it's often difficult to know what *is* best. In pregnancy and parenthood, there can be such pressure to strive tirelessly in our own effort, to figure things out, and to keep pace with the rest of the world and its ever-changing opinions. The result can be a striving for perfectionism that cripples our hearts and minds, as we can never attain the perfection of the world.

Thankfully, God does not expect us to parent our children alone. In Isaiah 40, God is speaking comfort and hope to the exiled Israelites in Babylonian captivity. God's power and sovereignty are on display, contrasted with the fleeting and frail nature of humans and nations. However, amid these descriptions of God's might, Isaiah depicts God as a gentle shepherd. His great strength, authority, and sovereignty do not prevent Him from also being kind, gentle, and compassionate to those who straggle behind with little ones.

Isaiah 40 reminds us to look up and see God's power and wisdom over the world. He alone is perfect, eternal, and wise. What we see here on earth is a vapor that will be gone tomorrow. In the perspective of eternity, whether you choose to get an epidural, use cloth diapers, eat only organic food, or breastfeed until age three are all such fleeting matters. The world pushes us to take sides and to do it quickly, but Isaiah calls us to look up and see that God is sovereign over all.

This high and powerful God carries you like a gentle shepherd. He leads you tenderly because He loves you and your young ones. Unlike the world, He is not pushing you to be perfect in motherhood. He wants you to look up and see that He is carrying you in His arms. Here is a sovereign, powerful God, who in that power is also gentle and merciful to those who have babies. As you carry your baby, in your womb now and in your arms later, take courage because He is carrying you.

A LITTLE PRAYER FOR YOU

Mighty God, turn my strivings for perfection into a
striving after You. I lay down my scrambling ambition
and my hustling nature and my want for perfection.
I want to depend wholly on You, be carried by You,
and know what it is to be gently led by You.

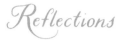

Reflections

What emotions do you feel when you imagine being
carried by God as a shepherd carries a lamb,
especially in this season of your life?

WEEK
21

Your baby is about 7 inches from crown to rump, though your provider may begin measuring from head to toe, in which case your baby is about 10½ inches long. Their eyes can detect light, though their eyelids will remain fused shut for a few more weeks, and you might feel the baby respond with kicks if you shine a flashlight on your belly. As your baby grows, your aches and discomforts might also increase, including heartburn, a stretching ligament pain, or leg cramps. Remember that God's grace is available to you as you experience these growing pains of pregnancy.

The grace of our Lord was poured out on me abundantly, along with the faith and love that are in Christ Jesus.

1 Timothy 1:14

GOD'S GRACE IN BIRTH

Many of us have in our minds the "correct" way to do things: Toilet paper should go over the roll, not under. Peanut butter should be creamy, not chunky. Toothpaste should be squeezed from the bottom of the tube up, not haphazardly from the middle. Dishes should be washed right after dinner, not left until the next morning.

We do this in childbirth, too. Some women feel strongly that the "right" way to give birth is completely drug free, at home rather than in a hospital, and with as little medical intervention as possible. Others want the hospital, doctors, as much pain relief as they are allowed, and the feeling of safety they get with medical instruments surrounding them. Other birth plans may be somewhere in between these two ends of the spectrum. It's easy to begin idolizing a birth plan, holding so tightly to it that any other kind of birth seems wrong or imperfect.

Every woman has her birth preferences, and that's good! It's better to be able to articulate those wishes rather than have an aimless approach. But as you begin making your birth plan, think of how you might cope if something were to throw off your expectations. If you plan to get an epidural as quickly as possible, what if you labor too quickly to get one? For a home birther, what if there are complications and you have to be taken to the hospital? Every pregnancy and birth is different and can suddenly take an unexpected turn. But a change in your birth plan isn't a cause for fear—it's an opportunity for God to pour His grace on you.

In his letter to Timothy, Paul explains how, even though he was a violent blasphemer before his Damascus Road experience, the Lord still lavished grace on him. This grace was not dependent on Paul's good works, his zealous heart, or his scholarly mind but simply because of Jesus' love for Paul.

In childbirth, you do not have to perform perfectly or make certain choices for God's grace to be poured out abundantly on you. His grace is already there for you. If your highly researched plans go sideways, Jesus will be there to extend grace for healing and learning more about Him. Ask for His wisdom as you research and take birthing classes. But instead of holding on to the "perfect" birth plan, pursue knowing Jesus more fiercely through your experiences.

A LITTLE PRAYER FOR YOU

Lord, I seek Your wisdom for the decisions I need to make about birth. Help me not to pursue the perfect birth but to pursue You through birth. Please pour Your grace on me throughout this pregnancy and birth. I want to know You more.

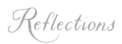

Reflections

What is your idea of the "right" kind of birth, and how might you feel if things don't go as planned?

_____

_____

_____

_____

_____

_____

_____

_____

_____

_____

_____

_____

_____

_____

_____

_____

_____

_____

Your baby is about 11 inches long, and their taste buds have developed so that they can detect in the amniotic fluid the flavors of what you've eaten. Their ears are also picking up your voice, music, and other sounds, so if you haven't begun talking to your baby, now is a good time! You might be starting to daydream about what this little person will look like and whether you can decipher their temperament from how they respond to your gentle pats. As you consider your baby's personality, think about who you are becoming as you grow as a mother.

So then, just as you received Christ Jesus as Lord, continue to live your lives in him, rooted and built up in him, strengthened in the faith as you were taught, and overflowing with thankfulness.

Colossians 2:6–7

A FIRM IDENTITY IN CHRIST

Different seasons of pregnancy and motherhood can challenge your sense of identity. Your sense of who you are might be wrapped up in the roles that you play in various areas of your life, and adding a new little life to the mix can shift those roles dramatically. You may truly rejoice at this shift but at the same time feel unsettled. These changes are a normal part of life—they'll crop up again as your children go off to kindergarten, start to drive, and leave home to strike out on their own.

In his letter to the Colossians, Paul uses the image of a plant to describe life in Christ. Believers are "rooted and built up" in Christ, both anchored to Him as their foundation and growing up into the wind, storms, and sunshine with His strength. In Christ, believers find who they truly are, as their whole lives become defined by His work and not their own. This rootedness in Christ results in an overflowing abundance of gratitude that spills out in all circumstances.

Your roles may be changing, but your identity is firm: you are in Christ, united with Him by His strength and stability. This sense of self holds fast in every stage and season of life, every loss and every gain. It can never be shifted or shaken, and it is something the world can never provide. Your identity is in Christ and in what He has done to make you belong to God.

Living in the reality of your true self can lead to a deeper sense of thankfulness and joy. You are a recipient of God's grace not because of anything you have accomplished—including your pregnancy or motherhood—but because of what Christ has done for us. Those who find all of who they are in Jesus alone, and not in themselves, will find freedom.

You might spend some time this week recounting your journey with Christ. Make a list of what you are grateful for in your union with Jesus. Pregnancy is a time to rejoice as a recipient of God's good gift to you of this baby and in the experience of bringing new life into the world. Hang up your list as a visual reminder of all that God has given to you in Christ and in the testimony of how He has sustained you.

A LITTLE PRAYER FOR YOU

Lord Jesus, thank You for coming after me, for saving me, and for sustaining me through all the changes of life. I'm grateful that my identity is in You, not in anything else. Help me anchor myself to that truth and to let it fill me to overflowing with gratitude.

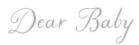

Dear Baby

Write a letter to your baby describing your story of how you came to faith in Christ and how you have been strengthened in that identity over the years.

WEEK
23

At over a pound in weight and almost 12 inches in length, your little one is growing rapidly! Their nervous system is working hard at developing reflexes, and now your baby can grab their own ears and nose. You may be experiencing swelling in your hands and ankles. Be sure to drink plenty of water to combat this, and consider storing any rings you wear until after pregnancy if your fingers are getting puffy. As you rely on your health-care provider to attend to your physical well-being, meditate on God's provision of spiritual care for you and your baby.

You brought me out of the womb; you made me trust in you, even at my mother's breast. From birth I was cast on you; from my mother's womb you have been my God. Psalm 22:9–10

HOLY MIDWIFE

In America, it is more common to see an obstetrician than a midwife for maternity needs, but in many countries, midwives are still preferred. For the ancient Israelites, midwives were trained women in the community who offered medical care and emotional comfort to women as they gave birth. Every culture has its birth traditions, and in Israel, midwives were the keepers of the knowledge that helps babies come safely into the world. After birth, midwives would also help mothers learn to breastfeed and to adjust to the realities of life with a little one.

David, as he wrote his Psalms, may have surprised his audience by describing God as a midwife. The same way a midwife might be the first person to catch an infant, God was close to David in the earliest moments of his life. Whereas a midwife would "cast" the baby to the mother's breast, David says he was cast on God from birth. David speaks of God as a nurturing birth worker who is present in an infant's life right from the beginning.

In the first months of a baby's life, deep trust is developed through their experience with their mother. They feel hunger, and when they make their needs known, those needs are met with milk and their mother's comforting warmth and loving arms. Did you know that the very act of feeding your child (whether by breast or by bottle) is an experience of expanding your baby's trust in you? When we are needy and someone fulfills that need faithfully, we develop trust. In this same way, David remarks that he learned to trust God even as he nursed from his mother because God has been with him from the start of his life.

The image of God as a midwife is a tremendous reminder of God's nearness to us in life, particularly at the sacred moment of birth. God brought David out of his mother's womb, as He brought you out of your mother's womb and as He will bring your baby out of your womb. His presence is with your baby even now and will be with your baby their whole life. What an incredible thing that God could be using your baby's experience of being nestled in your body, being brought out safely from your body, and being nurtured by you to draw your child into a trusting relationship with Him.

A LITTLE PRAYER FOR YOU

God, thank You for being with me in life and for being with my baby in the same way. Draw me into a deeper confidence in You, and develop even now a trust for You in my baby's little heart.

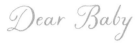

Dear Baby

Write a letter to your baby telling a story
from your life that demonstrates what it means
to trust and be cast upon God.

_____

_____

_____

_____

_____

_____

_____

_____

_____

_____

_____

_____

_____

_____

_____

_____

_____

_____

WEEK
24

Your baby is plumping up with sweet baby fat this week, and their brain is starting to form thoughts and memories similar to a newborn's. Your baby's lungs should also be fully formed though not quite ready to take those first breaths. During this phase of pregnancy, many women experience changes in their skin's pigmentation or get dry, itchy stretch marks. Sunscreen and moisturizer can help, and rubbing them in can even become a little game between you and your baby. As you feel those tumbles and hiccups, your anticipation to see and hold your baby grows into a joyful yearning.

We wait in hope for the Lord; he is our help and our shield. In him our hearts rejoice, for we trust in his holy name. May your unfailing love be with us, Lord, even as we put our hope in you.

Psalm 33:20–22

ACTIVELY WAITING

Your anticipation is growing to meet your little one, and it can be both challenging and exciting to be in such a season of waiting. In fact, much of pregnancy seems to involve that state of in-between: waiting to become pregnant, waiting to find out the results of a pregnancy test, waiting for symptoms to give way to relief, waiting for labor to begin (and end!), and waiting to hold your baby in your arms. The whole concept of "expecting" is loaded with longing for what lies in the future.

So much of life with God also involves waiting. The Israelites awaited deliverance from slavery in Egypt for over 400 years. They longed for a return from exile back to the Promised Land, then waited in anticipation for the Messiah, who would rescue them from spiritual exile. Even now, we await Jesus' return and the resurrection of our bodies. Waiting on the Lord is a frequent motif throughout Scripture and one we participate in with all God's people throughout history.

The Psalms perfectly express this feeling of anticipation and longing. The Psalmist writes that as we wait, we learn to trust God with our whole lives because He alone is our help. Our experience with God in these moments of waiting and fulfillment builds our confidence in Him as the ultimate promise keeper. As you wait in your pregnancy, you join the long story of the people of God who have waited and longed for God to deliver His promises. As they waited and as you wait, God teaches patience and joy along the way.

But we don't have to wait passively. Rejoice in the Lord during your waiting because you know that God is faithful and has good things planned for you. Because your hope is in God and not in what you wait for, you can rejoice right now, even before you receive what your heart longs for. Celebration should be a huge part of the Christian life, and you certainly have much to celebrate right now! Take time this week to express your joy in anticipation to the Lord and to others and to explore what He is teaching you in this time of waiting. As the Psalmist says, His unfailing love is with you as you place your hope in Him.

A LITTLE PRAYER FOR YOU

Jesus, thank You for this season of waiting that teaches me to long for You and to trust You in the waiting. Grow my patience and my faith as I look forward to my baby's birth, and help me rest in Your long history of faithfulness that endures forever.

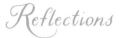

Reflections

In past seasons of waiting or anticipation,
how did you see the Lord grow you, and how
can you see His work in you now?

_____

_____

_____

_____

_____

_____

_____

_____

_____

_____

_____

_____

_____

_____

_____

_____

_____

_____

Your baby is about 13 inches long and one and a half pounds in weight. This week, to practice breathing after birth, their tiny nostrils will unseal and your baby will begin inhaling and exhaling amniotic fluid. You may find sleeping more of a struggle these days, as your baby often will be awake and active as soon as you lie down. Your walking motions during the day are lulling them to sleep, so they are raring to go when you relax at bedtime! Even as you struggle with sleep deprivation, reflect on and rest in the peace that God offers His people.

You will keep in perfect peace those whose minds are steadfast, because they trust in you. Trust in the Lord forever, for the Lord, the Lord himself, is the Rock eternal. Isaiah 26:3–4

GOD'S FOREVER PRESENCE

As your belly grows bigger, many activities will become uncomfortable, increasingly difficult, or even unsafe for you. If this is your first baby, you may also notice a subtle shift in your kid-free friend groups as you make the transition to parenthood. Invitations may not be extended to you for long hikes, sushi night, or an afternoon at the local theme park. Even though you know it's not safe for you to do those things, it's difficult not to feel twinges of loneliness, as if motherhood means that you've given up all the fun activities you used to do.

Isaiah promises that when we trust in the Lord and keep our minds steadfast, the Lord will keep us in perfect peace. Keeping your mind steadfast is difficult when things are changing quickly, and pregnancy hormones don't help the situation. Reading Scripture each morning can redirect lonely thoughts to the peaceful presence of God by washing your mind in the truth. When you receive love and truth from the Lord early each day, it can help you interpret the actions of others more clearly throughout the rest of your day. The Lord is our steady and eternal Rock, a firm foundation far more trustworthy than our emotions.

It is also important to communicate to your loved ones that you'd like to be included in some way when they do activities. Telling them how you're feeling can help them be sensitive to what you're going through. Let them know that even if you have to turn down an invitation, you want to be considered. Odds are, they miss you too and may be willing to consider more creative ways to include you or to enjoy a different, new activity with you during this season. Talking through this can result in enriching your friendships rather than endangering them.

While your life is changing, remind yourself that new adventures are ahead! Begin listing things you want to do with your child—where you want to travel someday, games and family traditions you want to incorporate, and skills you want to teach your child. Parenthood means that you will be gaining new adventures and memories with your growing family. Think of how fun it will be to swim with your child or travel on an airplane for the first time. Through every season, you can trust the Lord to be with you and that He desires good things for you.

A LITTLE PRAYER FOR YOU

Father God, thank You that You are always with me. Be near in my loneliness and when I feel left out. Please give me peace and keep my mind steadfast, and help me to trust You in all things as my Rock eternal.

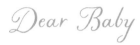

Dear Baby

Write a letter to your baby about the things you really look
forward to doing together.

At 14 inches and two pounds, your baby is filling out what used to be wrinkly skin to become a cute little chunk. This week, they will open their eyelids and begin to blink. If you have an ultrasound soon, you might catch your baby sucking their thumb or grabbing their toes, because they are becoming very skilled with their hands. The experiences you are having with your baby—their responses to sound or light, hiccups, or rolling over—may lead you to a more acute understanding of worship and joy as you marvel at God's creation within you.

"You are worthy, our Lord and God, to receive glory and honor and power, for you created all things, and by your will they were created and have their being." Revelation 4:11

WORTHY OF WORSHIP

If only we could see what the angels see, what all heaven experiences right now: God's full glory on display—brilliant colors, flashes of lightning, His thunderous voice, and an indescribable scene that would bring anyone to their knees in awe. The book of Revelation gives us a glimpse of this reality—the true reality—of God's worth, glory, and power, even as the earth below churns in its temporary troubles.

When we worship, we connect with this true and present reality, and we look forward to our full experience of worship alongside angels and saints before God's throne. Pregnancy may lead you to new depths of worship and awe for what God graciously does in you. It truly is a wonder to feel the movement of new life within your own body, knowing that this baby is being created by God and will someday soon be a separate person outside of your body. The joy and new love you experience in pregnancy can be an experience that draws you into deeper worship of the only One who could have ever designed such a miracle.

Not all worship is singing, but music engages our hearts, emotions, and bodies in a way that other forms of worship never could. You may even be at an advantage as a pregnant woman, as your hormones can heighten your sense of emotion. Our God gave us our emotions to reflect Him—a being who experiences love, joy, anger, compassion, jealousy, and sadness. Our emotions can lead us *toward* Him.

You might create a worship playlist to listen to on walks, while cleaning the kitchen, or as you're getting ready in the morning. Just as it's important to soak your mind in the truth of the Bible, it's important to soak your heart in worship of God. In worship, you can express your gratitude, joy, or sadness to Him with true authenticity. The music can move you into deep thankfulness and exaltation to Him for His works. Read the book of Revelation this week, looking for the eruptions of worship and the descriptions of God in His splendor. Then, think of the ways you can worship and praise God in your day-to-day activities. Worship helps align your heart with the reality that our powerful God is worthy of all glory and praise and allows you to participate in that reality, even now.

A LITTLE PRAYER FOR YOU

Creator God, the works of Your hands are incredible, and I'm so thankful that I get to experience and participate in Your creation in a new way. Cultivate in me a heart of praise and worship that exalts You for who You are— magnificent, good, and beyond comprehension.

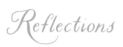

Reflections

Spend some time this week meditating on God's creative power, and journal some of the things you want to praise Him for.

WEEK
27

You are probably feeling your baby a lot these days as they kick, punch, tumble, and flip! These movements will slow down in intensity in the coming weeks as their quarters become more cramped, but these movements are a great sign that your baby is working out those muscles and nerves. As your second trimester draws to a close, you may be thinking more about the big event coming: childbirth! You have a lot of decisions to consider when it comes to birth and postpartum, but God is ready to provide the wisdom you're desperately seeking if you ask Him.

If any of you lacks wisdom, you should ask God, who gives generously to all without finding fault, and it will be given to you. James 1:5

MAKING DECISIONS

Congratulations! You're heading into your third trimester next week, and you'll soon hold this sweet baby in your arms. Before then, however, there are a lot of decisions to make. Have you started your birth and postpartum plans yet?

Some things you might be considering are how you'll manage contractions and discomfort, who will be present with you at the birth, how you want to feed your baby, what diapers your baby should wear, and where your baby will sleep. As you research each of your options, it's easy to become overwhelmed with the number of choices there are to make just in childbirth alone. There are good online tools and pregnancy books for creating a birth plan, and talking with your health-care provider or birth doula can be a great way of determining what is important to you.

But more important than researching and interviewing experts is cultivating a habit of asking God for wisdom in even the little decisions. The book of James reminds us that whenever we need wisdom, we can and should ask God because He gives it generously. Moreover, James says that believers should ask with a heart that *expects* God to answer them. There is no question too small or too big for God to answer, and He wants you to allow Him into this process of decision-making because He cares for you.

Your prayer to Him can be as simple as "Jesus, help!" It's astonishing how often we depend on our own wisdom and our own methods for gaining wisdom without ever asking God—the source of all wisdom. As you prepare for childbirth and parenthood, in any situation, you can come boldly to God's throne and cry out, "Jesus, help!" He's there waiting to help you by providing you the wisdom you need.

Parenting grows us in wisdom, and the Lord loves to grow our dependence upon Him as we come up against big decisions. The older our children get, the more complex decisions become, yet remember that no decision is too big for God. Have faith that when you ask for wisdom, He is waiting to generously give you what you need.

A LITTLE PRAYER FOR YOU

God, these decisions feel too much for me at times.
I need Your wisdom. Please guide me as I learn
from others, research, and make plans. Help me
walk confidently into the future, knowing that I
follow You and that You will never leave me.

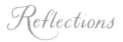

Reflections

Write out prayers to God for wisdom over
the decisions that loom ahead of you.

BIBLE STORIES TO READ ALOUD NOW

Talking to the baby in your belly might seem like a silly, one-sided conversation, but studies have shown that babies can begin to learn language even from inside the womb. Babies are attuned to the sound of their mother's voice, and talking to your unborn baby can help you develop a strong bond to the little one you can't yet see.

One way of fostering this bond is to begin reading Bible stories to your baby. You might consider establishing a bedtime routine of telling your child Bible stories and praying over them, starting now. Many times, mothers find that the stories they read to their child in the womb are the ones that their babies love most after birth. Reading these stories will show your child how much you love God and will help foster a love of God in their own life.

There are many good, beautifully illustrated children's storybooks for infants, toddlers, and preschoolers to help you teach the Bible to your child, including the ones recommended below:

The Jesus Storybook Bible: Every Story Whispers His Name by Sally Lloyd-Jones

The Beginner's Bible: Timeless Children's Stories

The Complete Illustrated

Children's Bible by Janice Emmerson

Children's Bible Stories for Bedtime: Stories to Grow in Faith and Love by Julie Lavender

PASTE
PHOTO
HERE

BUMP PHOTO

PASTE
PHOTO
HERE

BABY'S NURSERY

IN GOD'S HANDS

You're in the home stretch! These final weeks of pregnancy may truly feel like a stretch as your belly expands farther than you thought it could, sleep seems more elusive, and you're filled with a longing for labor to finally begin. This trimester, you're probably thinking of all that you need to do to prepare for this new life coming your way: taking childbirth and breastfeeding classes, assembling cribs and bouncers, washing onesies, and stockpiling diapers—there's a lot to do! But through the frenzy, find peace in reading God's Word and studying the weekly devotions. These times will help you joyfully anticipate your baby's arrival.

Your little one has grown to 15 inches long, and according to a 2017 study published in *PLOS ONE*, babies at this stage of development can dream when they sleep. By this time, many babies have positioned themselves for birth with their head at the bottom of your abdomen. You can encourage this positioning by sitting up straight, leaning over a birth ball, or getting on your hands and knees rather than lounging back in a recliner. As practice contractions become more common for you, take those moments to breathe deeply and release yourself into God's affection for you, His child.

Yet to all who did receive him, to those who believed in his name, he gave the right to become children of God—children born not of natural descent, nor of human decision or a husband's will, but born of God. John 1:12–13

YOUR EXPANDING LOVE

As your child grows within you, your heart will seem to expand with deep love for them. You feel protective of this little person you've never seen, and you can't wait to see their face and drink in that precious baby smell. You look forward to hearing their little babbles, comforting them when they're scared, telling them stories at bedtime, or watching them play. There is so much to anticipate as a parent, so much joy ahead of you.

For many, parenthood is a profound relearning of God's heart for them. John writes that all who trust in Christ become children of God. Elsewhere, Biblical writers describe this relationship in terms of adoption, from slaves of sin to children of God. But John prefers the analogy of birth: as God's children, we are born of God into His family.

As His children, even though our Father is the king of the universe, we get to come to Him anytime, without having to dress ourselves up first. Just as your toddler will come to you with skinned knees and a tearstained face while you're talking on the phone, we can come to our Father with all our chaos and messes anytime. Just as your child brings your heart joy in their attempts to imitate you, how much more do your fumbling attempts to imitate Christ bring joy to God! Just as you will give your child nourishing food, clean water, a safe place to sleep, and a loving hug, so will your Father provide everything you need. Just as you do these things because you love your child no matter their behavior, so does your heavenly Father love you generously apart from your behavior.

We often relate to God as employees: we learn the rules, we obey them, and we worry about being fired when we fail. But God invites you to be His child, and if you are in Christ, you are part of the family—your place is secure; you are loved and cherished. Because you are so loved, you should want to please your good Father and become more like Him as you grow—just as your children want to please you because you love them. This is why the analogy of family in the Christian life is so powerful. It is a picture of unearned favor, belonging, and the flourishing life that emerges from God's love.

A LITTLE PRAYER FOR YOU

Father, thank You for choosing me to be Your child, welcoming me into Your family, and giving me all the rights that come with it. I pray that my experience of parenting will help me more completely understand the love and belonging that I have in You.

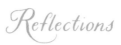

Reflections

What does being born into God's family mean to you, and how can your own parenting mirror God's parenting of you?

WEEK

29

This week marks an important point in your baby's development because this is the week that their lungs make surfactant, a substance that keeps their lungs inflated after birth. Because of this substance, if they were born now, they would need less intensive medical treatment than babies born before this week. At two and a half pounds, your baby is starting to fill up your abdomen. You may find that your fatigue returns in the next few weeks along with other unpleasant symptoms. Take heart—God gives strength to those who feel weak and can empower you to endure the weariness.

He gives strength to the weary and increases the power of the weak . . . but those who hope in the Lord will renew their strength. They will soar on wings like eagles; they will run and not grow weary, they will walk and not be faint.

Isaiah 40:29, 31

HOPE IN THE LORD

Right now, you're probably feeling pretty good, especially compared with the marathon you endured during the first trimester. Your body's strength and power to nourish new life is a marvel, and some women feel a sense of boundlessness in what they can do. But the "limitless" message will likely ring less true in the coming weeks as you come face-to-face with your very real limitations and exhaustion. Prepare your heart now for the weariness ahead, and strengthen your hope in the Lord so that it holds firm when exhaustion sets in.

Pregnancy can make you weary in all kinds of ways. As your baby grows heavier over the next few months, physical fatigue will grow as well. You may find it harder to sleep as your little one parties through the night. Your mind might be drained from all the decisions you need to make to prepare for childbirth and the long road of parenting afterward. Perhaps you feel dragged down from other situations in your life that are compounded by pregnancy hormones and the rapid changes your body and life are making.

When you feel weary, you might lean upon something that makes you feel more secure and stable, something you can place your hope in. This could be a number of things: birth classes that promise easier labor, parenting methods that assure well-behaved kids, products that promise full nights of sleep or quiet newborns. None of these is bad—intentional planning and thoughtfulness in your approach to parenting is recommended. But none of these is a sure foundation of hope. None renews our strength like the Lord can.

Relying on your own inner resources will only leave you more exhausted and hopeless, but leaning on the Lord will give you strength and peace for the days ahead. What does hoping in the Lord look like? It's turning to God in prayer for your needs. It's asking for help when you can't keep up with all you need to do. It's renewing your mind in truth by reading your Bible and learning from God about how He is trustworthy and how you can come to Him for anything. For those who feel weak and weary, the Lord offers His strength and power. This weakness that you feel should drive you to seek out power and help from God, your true and sure source of hope.

A LITTLE PRAYER FOR YOU

Lord, I need Your strength in my weakness. Would You help me turn to You rather than to my own resources and place my hope only in You? Help me accept my limited nature and depend on Your grace alone.

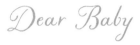

Dear Baby

Write a letter to your baby sharing what difficulties you've faced in this pregnancy and where you have seen the Lord giving you strength.

_____

_____

_____

_____

_____

_____

_____

_____

_____

_____

_____

_____

_____

_____

_____

_____

_____

_____

_____

_____

At 16 inches and three pounds, your little one is beginning to run out of room for their tumbling gymnastics routines. Your baby will begin putting on about half a pound of weight per week from now on, so you may find that your body begins to demand more nutrition as well. Food may taste especially delicious—enjoy it! Your breasts also may begin leaking small amounts of milk as they gear up for nourishing your baby in a new way. It's incredible how God designed your body and your heart to meet your baby's needs, both before and after birth.

Just as a nursing mother cares for her children, so we cared for you. Because we loved you so much, we were delighted to share with you not only the gospel of God but our lives as well.

1 Thessalonians 2:7b–8

MATERNAL INSTINCTS

There are lots of women who are "maternal" by nature: They've always been drawn to children, wanted to be mothers, and loved playing with kids or babysitting them as teenagers. But other women may feel intimidated by bringing a new baby into this world. Some fear they won't know what to do, won't understand their children's cries, or won't figure out how to raise their children in the ways of the Lord. They may even have vivid dreams during pregnancy about leaving the baby alone at home or at the store. What if that maternal instinct never comes and they aren't able to care for their baby?

When Paul, Silas, and Timothy wrote their letter to the Thessalonian church, they described their care and affection for their church community as both nursing mothers and encouraging fathers. This deep love drove them to work hard and even suffer on the church's behalf—a difficult road that many parents understand and would do a million times over for their beloved children.

Likewise, the strong biological drive to care for newborns—whether you're already feeling it or it comes further down the road—is something that's hard to deny. God has designed a mother's body so that her hormones drive her to meet her child's needs. Oxytocin, the "love hormone" that floods a woman's body during childbirth and when breastfeeding, fills her with feelings of warmth, affection, and elation toward her baby. God is bonding you to your baby, both in your body and in your heart, in a special way that will enable you to care for your child.

Even those who do not consider themselves maternal toward others' children will find themselves transformed into caring and nurturing mothers with deeply ingrained instincts toward their own babies. This experience often leads them to eventually exhibit motherly love toward others' children as well as their own. You may not always know what to do in a given situation, but in these moments, pray for wisdom and seek out help. God gives us our communities and churches and families, made up of many mothers seeking wisdom, for just this purpose. Learning how to mother will come *as* you mother, and you can trust the instincts and the other mothers in your community and church that God has given to help you.

A LITTLE PRAYER FOR YOU

God, I trust that You have given me this child, knowing
that I will be able to mother them in Your strength
and as a reflection of how You care for Your children.
Grow in me an attentiveness to You and to my baby.

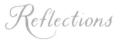

Reflections

What parts of motherhood are you worried
you will have no maternal instincts for?

Your baby is working on their breathing by practicing the inhale-exhale movements they'll need in just a few more weeks. Your baby's facial expressions can show what they feel now, thanks to fine-tuned muscular movements. If you were to see your baby on a 4D ultrasound, which shows highly detailed images and movements, you might see your little one smile or frown! It's unbelievable to think that God Himself became human and was nestled in the womb of Mary, as your baby is in your womb now. What a sacred space childbearing is, where heaven and earth meet in Christ!

"Therefore the Lord himself will give you a sign:
The virgin will conceive and give birth to a son,
and will call him Immanuel." Isaiah 7:14

GOD WITH US

One of the most profound names for Jesus is Immanuel, meaning "God with us." For millennia, God spoke through prophets to His people. He spoke from thunderous clouds, burning bushes, bizarre dreams, and blazing mountains. He gave them holy spaces—the tabernacle and then the temple—so they could draw near to Him in ways that wouldn't destroy them in the presence of His holiness. Finally, He Himself came near. In Jesus, all the fullness of God and true humanity were united in a mysterious and unexpected way: in a baby.

For centuries, the Jews had been looking for a Messiah, the Anointed One who would rescue them from their political oppressors and from spiritual exile. The Messiah would come in power, establish His kingdom, and vindicate Israel among all her enemies. While the Jews looked for a fierce warrior king, Jesus was born quietly in a tiny village to an impoverished couple. Though there were angelic proclamations and heavenly choirs singing over His birth, Jesus was a true baby who experienced true human birth. Jesus, as God in the flesh, became the new temple: the place where heaven and earth met, the only place that could not be overthrown by any powers of the world. They tried, and He rose three days later! In Christ, humanity can now approach God in holiness in any place.

God accomplished this coming near through the most unlikely method: childbirth. Jesus' body grew and formed in Mary's womb, as your baby's body is doing now in yours. Through His birth, God Himself came into our mess. Birth is not clean and tidy, but God gave Himself over to the womb and birth canal for you and me. Truly, Immanuel is with us in all things. There is no place He will not go with and for us.

Birth is now a sacred space Jesus inhabits with us. He is a good High Priest because He has experienced the full scope of what it means to be human—what it means to be frail, hungry, poor, tempted, and small. Therefore, we can go before Him confidently with all our needs, knowing He understands it all. As your baby grows in your womb now, and as you experience childbirth soon, be encouraged that Immanuel—God with us— has already been in that space. His presence makes it all sacred, a place where heaven meets earth and where He meets us.

A LITTLE PRAYER FOR YOU

Jesus, thank You for coming near to us and for experiencing all of what it means to be human so that You could be our great High Priest. Thank You that we can come to You confidently, knowing that You have mercy and compassion on us.

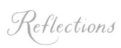

Reflections

What is significant to you about the incarnation—God made flesh—and how does it relate to your upcoming birth?

Much of the protective hair covering your baby's body has disappeared, and all their major organs (except their lungs) are fully operational! Your baby is around four pounds and 17 inches long. By this week, their startle reflex has developed, so if your baby hears a sudden loud noise, you may feel them react with strong movements! You may have begun walking with a waddle, but make sure you keep walking—gentle exercise will keep your muscles in shape for birth and postpartum. As your baby prepares for their entrance into the world, consider how you are preparing to guide your child through life with God.

Love the Lord your God with all your heart and with all your soul and with all your strength. These commandments that I give you today are to be on your hearts. Impress them on your children. Deuteronomy 6:5–7a

A LASTING LEGACY

As you bring your child into this world, you may be considering the kind of parent you will be and what legacy you want to leave for your child. Children are often drawn into whatever their parents love and do. Some families are wild fans of a particular sports team; other families spend hours reading books together; and some are active outdoors and spend significant time hiking, camping, or riding bikes. Many of the things you teach your children to love will simply come from your heart—they will see you enjoy a particular thing and will absorb a love for it too.

As a parent, you will have tremendous influence over your children, and what you teach them to value—education, good food, exercise—may stay with your family for generations. Moses knew the weight of a parent's legacy and teaching, and in his final sermon to the Israelites before crossing into the Promised Land, he impressed parents with the magnitude of their influence. Above all else, Moses encouraged them to love God with their whole selves and to let that love pervade their lives in obedience to God. This would provide a daily example to the children living in their household.

Further, Moses commanded them to always teach their children about God—while sitting at home, putting kids to bed, or walking around town. As you go about daily life—washing dishes, folding laundry, grocery shopping—every moment is a potential opportunity to teach your children how to love God and to walk with Him.

Loving God goes beyond taking your children to church on Sundays, though that's certainly one piece of it. Your child will be with you the other six days as well. Consider what your child will see and hear on those other days. Will they see you shoveling the snow from the elderly neighbor's driveway? Will they hear you speaking kind words about people who exasperate you? Will they stumble out of bed each morning to find you with your Bible open and coming to the Lord in prayer? The most profound legacy you can leave your child is one that directs them toward loving the Lord with all their heart, soul, and strength. Like the other things you love, it may be "caught" more than it is taught.

A LITTLE PRAYER FOR YOU

Lord God, I want to be a parent who teaches my
child Your ways and guides them in Your truth.
Help me love You with all that I am, and give me
wisdom to faithfully teach Your ways to my child.

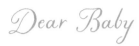

Dear Baby

Write a letter to your baby about how you want to intentionally teach and guide them toward life in the Lord.

Your baby's immune system is up and running this week, ready to defend your baby outside the womb, though they still receive protective antibodies from your body through the placenta. Your little one has grown fingernails and toenails, which may already need to be clipped at birth. As your baby continues to pack on the pounds, you might find that there is less room for your lungs to catch a good breath. Give yourself grace to move more slowly and to take breaks. Pray for the Lord to give you perseverance in these last weeks of pregnancy as your fatigue returns in full force.

For everything that was written in the past was written to teach us, so that through the endurance taught in the Scriptures and the encouragement they provide we might have hope.

Romans 15:4

FAITHFUL ENDURANCE

While there's much to enjoy about pregnancy, many women find that their last several weeks feel more like a feat of both physical and emotional endurance. Thankfully, there are many stories in the Bible that can encourage and inspire us in various seasons and circumstances—including these last weeks of pregnancy.

In his letter to the Romans, Paul encourages the church to look to the past as recorded in the Bible for examples of endurance. Paul offers David, who experienced many trials in his walk with the Lord, as one example of not only perseverance but also God's faithfulness in the midst of trying circumstances. Stories are powerful because of their ability to connect readers with truths in profound ways. The Bible is largely made up of stories. These narratives invite us into the plot, and they help us see what the characters can't always see: that God is the writer of these stories, and He is moving the story toward His purposes.

Stories of God's people can encourage us toward more faithful obedience in our lives. For decades, Sarah waited in a fumbling faith for God to fulfill His promises for her to become pregnant and provide an heir. Likewise, Daniel served king after king in captivity but looked to the one true King over all creation for his strength. Which stories of endurance from the Bible are especially encouraging to you in this current season?

The ultimate story of endurance, of course, is of Jesus' death on the cross and His resurrection to bring wholeness back to this world and defeat death. Jesus knows what it means to labor and groan so that new life can emerge from darkness. He knows what it is to give His body over for love of someone else. You can learn to run long and hard races alongside Jesus because He ran long, hard races. If pregnancy is beginning to feel like a feat of endurance for you, take hope and encouragement that you are joining the long story of the perseverance of God's people.

This week, ask God to give you a story from Scripture that will speak to your current circumstances. Read it carefully and prayerfully, expecting Him to speak to you through that story, and make notes about what gives you hope and encouragement and spurs you on toward endurance in Christ.

A LITTLE PRAYER FOR YOU

Jesus, please give me Your endurance in these
last weeks of pregnancy. Help me run this race
alongside You with joy and hope, knowing that the
finish line is coming soon. Teach me through this
pregnancy how to endure other long races in life.

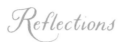

Reflections

Which parts of pregnancy feel like a feat of endurance right now, and what stories encourage you toward faithful endurance?

_____

_____

_____

_____

_____

_____

_____

_____

_____

_____

_____

_____

_____

_____

_____

_____

_____

_____

_____

Your uterus is preparing for birth with practice contractions called Braxton-Hicks, and if this isn't your first baby, they might be stronger than you remember. Your baby is getting close to their birth size at around five pounds in weight and 18 inches long. Your discomfort is likely increasing these days, which is actually a good thing—most women end up longing for labor by the end of pregnancy rather than fearing it, as they might have in earlier weeks! As you think ahead to childbirth, marvel at the ways God has designed your body for such an amazing physical feat.

Come, let us bow down in worship, let us kneel before the Lord our Maker; for he is our God and we are the people of his pasture, the flock under his care. Psalm 95:6–7

YOUR BODY'S HOLY DESIGN

As their baby grows each week, many women begin to wonder how they could possibly give birth. Pushing the baby out seems like an impossible physical task! In reality, though, God is a good creator and designer, and He has made your body to do this incredible work. Most mothers look back on their childbirth experiences—of all kinds—and marvel at how strong their bodies were and how amazed they are that they were able to do such a thing. Ask any mother about her birth story, and she will likely give you a long, detailed, and perhaps emotional tale! Birth is a powerful experience precisely because of the seeming impossibility of it.

Even now, your body is preparing for birth. You might be tired of Braxton-Hicks contractions, but those are a sign that your uterus is strengthening itself for the big day ahead. For most athletic events, you are responsible for training and strengthening your body, but for birth, your uterus does it automatically. Your cervix holds your baby in and keeps them safe in your womb, and unless your body is ready for birth, even medical induction might not get the cervix to open! God also designed your birth canal to widen and stretch to precisely accommodate your baby's exit. How amazing it is that God created your body to know exactly how to prepare for and deliver your baby.

In labor, your body will respond to pain in incredible ways, like by producing oxytocin—the "love hormone." This hormone is a friend that helps you meet the next contraction and open your body to deliver the baby. It is possible that your body will need additional help in birth, whether that is Pitocin or a cesarean section. This is not a failure on your part; rather, it is an opportunity to grow in your trust in God. Trials are a time to be diligent in prayer and grounded in knowing that God is with you. Begin thinking today about how you can work with your body's natural design to labor in God's love. Trust in His design and marvel at the ways your body does this incredible work!

A LITTLE PRAYER FOR YOU

Creator God, thank You for Your good design of my body, which You have created to be able to give birth—an unbelievable feat! Give me courage and confidence in You as I approach labor, and replace all my fears with Your peace and Your abiding presence.

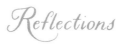

Reflections

Picture God in the delivery room with you. What does it mean to labor alongside Him, and what fears, plans, thoughts, and expectations can you entrust to Him?

Much of the developmental work of your baby's body is finished, and these next few weeks are all about gaining weight in preparation for birth. Your baby's movements will be less dramatic than before, but you'll still feel plenty of activity. You may feel there can be no more room for this child—they're already sitting on your bladder, pushing against your lungs, and leaving little room in your stomach for food! As your baby continues to fill out physically, pray about how you can "fill up" your child spiritually as they mimic you in the years to come.

Even if you had ten thousand guardians in Christ, you do not have many fathers, for in Christ Jesus I became your father through the gospel. Therefore I urge you to imitate me.

1 Corinthians 4:15–16

TINY IMITATORS

From their very first moments of life, newborns are constantly learning how to live in this world by mimicking the cues received from those who care for them. By two months old, they mirror the smiles given to them. By six months, they often begin copying the sounds they've been hearing from the womb and may even pronounce simple syllables. Preschoolers will pretend to drink coffee, work on computers, play with phones, and repeat anything they've seen adults doing. Ask any preschool teacher, and they could probably tell you a lot about the parents of the children they teach simply from how their children play!

It can be hilarious, sweet, or even embarrassing to see your mannerisms, words, and actions come from your little one. The brains of babies and young children absorb everything around them, and their observation skills are astounding. God has wired their brains to look to those around them and to imitate them. As such, having children is an intense discipleship opportunity for you!

The apostle Paul often urged churches and those he mentored to imitate him as a child imitates their parents. Paul modeled his own life after Jesus in his teachings, sufferings, humility, service, and care for others. Even for adults, it can be difficult to know how to live a godly life unless we have seen it ourselves. It's one thing to learn about abstract concepts, like sacrificially loving others. But it's more powerful and formative to see a person actually *being* sacrificially loving toward someone else. Imitating others teaches us how to live out complex and difficult ideas rather than merely believe them.

Seeing your child imitate you can be somewhat intimidating, but God doesn't expect you to be a perfect parent. Parenting is the ultimate learning experience—not a single person has it figured out beforehand—so don't allow shame or fear to weigh you down. Instead, trust that God will help you guide your child in His ways and accept the grace and forgiveness that God offers us all.

As a follower of Christ, what will you see your child mimic? Throughout the week, prayerfully consider if there are any areas of your life in which you need to change with the Spirit's help. Your child will witness your habits, passions, and treatment of others more intimately than the rest of the world does. You will then have the perfect opportunity to show your children the ways of God.

A LITTLE PRAYER FOR YOU

Lord, I thank You that You have created us to be
like You. Help me seek intimacy with You and to
walk with You in obedience and faithfulness as I
become someone that my child will someday imitate.
Help my child see and experience Jesus in me.

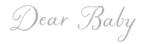

Dear Baby

Make some predictions! Tell your baby ways you think they might physically look like you and what character qualities you hope they will someday imitate.

Your baby's circulatory system is now fully developed and ready for life outside the womb. As your baby "drops" into your pelvis, you may get some relief this week, providing much more space to breathe and eat normally (but you may also find yourself heading to the bathroom more frequently as your baby squishes your bladder). For some, this "lightening" doesn't happen until labor begins. As your body works hard to create new life, reflect on the Biblical imagery of the new life that we have in Christ through His laboring—not our own.

Praise be to the God and Father of our Lord Jesus Christ! In his great mercy he has given us new birth into a living hope through the resurrection of Jesus Christ from the dead. 1 Peter 1:3

BIRTH: A PICTURE OF THE GOSPEL

One of the most profound metaphors of salvation in the New Testament is that of a second birth. John records a conversation between Jesus and Nicodemus, a member of the Jewish ruling council. Nicodemus had sneaked under the cover of night to ask Jesus about His difficult teachings. In answer, Jesus explained Nicodemus' need for an entirely new birth from God's Spirit to see the kingdom of God. Humanity doesn't need a solution here, a repair there—it needs an entirely new creation from God, a full overhaul and a complete remaking. Jesus initiated this transformation through His death and resurrection, and one day, all creation will be made new when Jesus returns.

The language of childbirth is significant for this process. In natural childbearing, an entirely new person is formed in the darkness of the mother's womb. Through the travail of the mother, the baby is born into the world through no effort of their own. A child is delivered and received into life through grace alone. There is nothing more precious than this new life, bought with trial, blood, and pain.

Jesus' death and resurrection bring an even more profound newness of life than birth does. It is only through His suffering on the cross, taking the evils and death of this world onto His physical body, that we gain new life. His labor, like a mother's, is done out of pure, fierce love and not for His own self. He brings His children from darkness to light and into new life through

His own sorrows. Further, the God who rebirths us is now our parent. What could signal this full remaking in Christ better than a newborn baby?

As His reborn children, we are to imitate Him as we were always intended to do before sin broke the intimacy between God and humanity. We are born into His family, gaining a security and an honor we could never have achieved for ourselves. With Him, we become the humans we were always intended to be.

As your body co-creates with God, consider the profound metaphor that childbirth is for the gospel. Consider the ways your pregnancy and childbirth experiences are a picture of what God does for us in Christ, and consider the living hope that we have because God has given us new life.

A LITTLE PRAYER FOR YOU

Jesus, I praise You for the way You have travailed
to give me new life in You. Thank You for making
me a new creation, brought from darkness into
light. Continue to teach me about Yourself through
my own experience of pregnancy and birth.

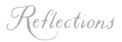

Reflections

Reflect on the profound ways that pregnancy, childbirth, and parenting can teach us about the gospel and what effect it has on you.

WEEK
37

Great news: Your baby is considered full-term this week! Healthy babies are born anywhere from 37 to 42 weeks' gestation, so think of your due date as more of a "due month." Babies vary greatly in weight during these last weeks, but most weigh around six pounds right now. You're likely feeling tired, uncomfortable, and ready for labor to begin. At the same time, you may be nervous about labor and dread its onset. God longs to give you peace in all situations, including childbirth. Challenge yourself to take hold of His peace this week as you prepare for the delivery room.

"Peace I leave with you; my peace I give you. I do not give to you as the world gives. Do not let your hearts be troubled and do not be afraid." John 14:27

PEACE IN LABOR

Pain serves a protective purpose in our bodies. It tells us to move away from a fire that scorches a finger or signals that something has gone wrong and you need medical attention. Pain in your back may tell you to rest your body or to sleep in another position. Pain doesn't feel good, but it's a good thing we feel it!

Most women do experience pain in childbirth for a number of reasons. The cervix can give a sharp twinge as it slowly opens, contractions may push your baby into uncomfortable positions, and parts of your body will be stretched in new ways. These are normal signals that something tremendous is happening, and in most cases, if you work with your body, helping it relax and open rather than fighting against it, you can actually reduce the amount of pain you perceive.

As a Christian, you know God gives "peace that surpasses understanding" to His people. He is a God who loves to rescue His people from fear and bless them with a sense of calm that no other thing in this world can give. Whether you labor for hours or have a cesarean, God is able to grant you peace as you bring this new little life into the world.

You may have images of childbirth in your mind absorbed from movies and television—mothers screaming through the whole ordeal, wild with fear and in constant pain. Most birth scenes are included in these dramas to add a sense of crisis and suspense rather than to accurately portray a real-life birth. But these aren't true births. Yes, the pressure and sensations are painful—there's no way to sugarcoat it—but each contraction lasts only a short amount of time. Most are less than a minute, with several minutes of rest in between! Use the breaks between contractions to relax your body and to hold fast to the inner serenity that God longs to give you in childbirth. Remember that God is there and His peace is available to you. He will bless you, calling you into love and not fear, and His presence is with you to calm and comfort you as you cry out to Him. As you labor, consider having a person in your support system read a few verses about God's peace to remind you of His never-ending comfort and help take your mind off the pain.

A LITTLE PRAYER FOR YOU

Lord Jesus, please bless me with Your abundant peace this week. Help me not to be afraid, and enable me to give over my worries to You. Surround me with a sense of Your love for me and my baby, and help me prepare my mind and body to receive Your peace in birth.

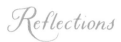

Reflections

What would it look like to be peaceful—in the power of Christ—as you give birth, and what are things you could do to give yourself over to His peace?

_____

_____

_____

_____

_____

_____

_____

_____

_____

_____

_____

_____

_____

_____

_____

_____

_____

_____

Your baby's lungs are fully developed and ready to take their first breaths after birth! As your little one continues to put on more weight in preparation for their entrance into the world, you are likely slowing down significantly this week. One of the great joys of pregnancy is that because your body is working so hard, everyone feels you deserve a nap, so take one if you are able! As you find your physical limitations increasing, rest in God's command for a Sabbath. He is not concerned with how much you get done but is a caring Father who wants you to rest in Him.

There remains, then, a Sabbath-rest for the people of God; for anyone who enters God's rest also rests from their works, just as God did from his.

Hebrews 4:9–10

HITTING YOUR LIMITS

Our culture tends to applaud overworking and busyness. We wear an invisible badge of honor if we are highly productive, work all hours, and never seem to have free time. Special praise may be given for overworking if it's ministry related, because we're doing "God's work" to utter exhaustion. Surely we are valuable if we are busy and act as if we had no limitations.

While it's admirable to work hard in the time God has given you, dipping into a compulsive pattern of overworking is not God's design for human flourishing. At creation, God Himself rested after six days of labor, setting a pattern for humanity to follow. The Sabbath—God's day of rest—was intended to be a holy day, set apart for God's glory and for humanity's good. Laws against collecting a harvest, cooking food, buying or selling, and even having slaves or animals do this work set boundaries around human productivity. One day a week, people were expected to accept their limitations and rest in God's grace and provision for them. This time was also to allow people's bodies to rest and recover in preparation for the next several days of work.

Sabbath, for many people, can be a difficult discipline as they lay down their need to control, provide, produce, and do. Resting one day per week, however, is an intentional entrusting of important things to God's sovereignty, care, and provision. It's a rebellion against the idea that work is a priority over being with God.

Sabbath is a set-apart day that belongs to God, and we should spend the day in His presence as set-apart people. This may include going to church, but that isn't the whole of it. Rest, play, and delight should be part of the rhythm of God's people, and this is no less true for you in pregnancy and motherhood—a season sometimes marked by exhaustion and never-ending work.

Begin praying now about setting boundaries in your family life around your work. How can you honor God's intended rhythms of work and rest as a mother so that you experience refreshment and delight in Him? As your body finds its very real limitations and slowness here at the end of pregnancy, consider how rhythms of rest are important not only for your body but also for your soul. What is something you can do today to rest in Him?

A LITTLE PRAYER FOR YOU

Sovereign God, You alone are limitless. I repent of my striving for control and productivity, for finding my worth in what I do rather than in You. Thank You for providing true rest in Jesus. Help me lay down my work regularly to honor and worship You, trusting Your provision.

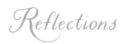

Reflections

Record your thoughts and prayers on resting in God,
especially as you approach new limitations in pregnancy.

_____

_____

_____

_____

_____

_____

_____

_____

_____

_____

_____

_____

_____

_____

_____

_____

_____

_____

_____

_____

Your baby has achieved their birth weight, and now it's just a waiting game for labor to begin! You may find that you get a surge of energy sometimes in these last few weeks, and suddenly, you see everything that needs to be cleaned, organized, or thrown out. Take full advantage of this nesting period, but be careful not to overdo it. Make sure you are familiar with the signs of labor, and have your bags ready to go! As you prepare your home for your new little one, begin preparing your heart for the new journey you're embarking on.

"He marked out their appointed times in history and the boundaries of their lands. God did this so that they would seek him and perhaps reach out for him and find him, though he is not far from any one of us." Acts 17:26b–27

THE JOYS OF NESTING

You're getting so close to your little one's arrival! As you wait with anticipation (and maybe some impatience!), you might find yourself in full-blown nesting mode. After weeks of feeling increasingly tired, you suddenly have a burst of motivation for assembling new furniture, stocking the freezer, doing laundry, organizing drawers, cleaning baseboards, and scrubbing tile grout. As your body prepares for labor, it sends signals to your brain that alert you to prepare your space for your new arrival.

Just as you ready your home to welcome your baby, God is also preparing a place for you and your baby. In his sermon to the Athenians in Acts, Paul states that when God created people, He set them in certain times and places. Where they are born, what family they are born into, which moment in history—all these details are mapped out by God so each person might seek God and find Him. God prepares the spaces and times for each of us, knowing that these details are our best option for coming to know Him.

The book of Esther tells a powerful story of a Jewish girl in exile who becomes queen to the most powerful king in the world at the time. When her people are threatened with genocide, her cousin urges her not to keep silent to spare her own life but to beg the king to spare her people. God placed her in that exact position during an exact moment in history to accomplish His purposes, and she used her position of influence with the king to save her people from destruction. Who knows but that you have become this child's mother for such a time as this?

God is sovereign over the timing of your pregnancy and the circumstances your child is being born into. What an encouragement that even if things are not "perfect," God is bringing this child into your family, at this time and place, so that your baby might reach out to God and find Him. Prepare your home and plan your meals as well as you are able, but most of all, prepare your heart for what the Lord is calling you into in this upcoming season of motherhood. Have faith to believe that God has called you to this new life.

A LITTLE PRAYER FOR YOU

God, thank You for Your care over the details of my life so that I would seek You and find You. Help me see the ways that You are doing this for my baby, and help me rise in Your strength to be the mother this baby needs.

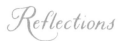

Reflections

Reflect on God's "boundary marking" that led you toward Him and how you can share that with your child so they can see God in their own life.

WEEK
40

About 70 percent of pregnant women have their babies by the end of week 40, so it's likely that you will meet your baby this week (if you haven't already!). If you find yourself heading into week 41 or 42, try not to despair! Your body is keeping your baby safe and sound until just the right time. Whenever you do go into labor or have your cesarean scheduled, one of the most important things for you to know is that God is with you, He delights in you, and He takes joy in your work to bring this baby into the world.

"The Lord your God is with you, the Mighty Warrior who saves. He will take great delight in you; in his love he will no longer rebuke you, but will rejoice over you with singing." Zephaniah 3:17

A LABOR OF LOVE

God takes joy in you as you labor and give birth. As a Christian, you don't have to come to birth afraid of the pain that you will endure. (Nor should you for one second have to subscribe to the idea that this is God's curse to all women.) Instead, you can see through the pain to the God who is with you through it all. The labor of birth is a wonderful opportunity to cling to God and allow Him to help you bring new life into this world.

You, indwelled by the Holy Spirit, are the object of His utter affection as you give birth. You are doing holy work in Christ, God-given work, self-sacrificing and loving work that mirrors what Jesus has done for you. He takes joy in you as you yield to Him all your fears and doubts, all your elation and wonder. He is pleased with you and longs for your good, even in labor, even if things don't go according to plan.

Today's verse describes God as a mighty warrior who saves and delights in us. All throughout Scripture, God's love is described as chasing down humans to restore them to His presence right from the first transgression. Even in the warnings of the prophets and in Israel's ejection from the Promised Land, God's judgment is couched in language of long-suffering, compassion, grief, and longing to restore. This self-sacrificing, loving God is the same God who is with you in labor.

When labor begins, don't fear the next contraction or the pain. God is a mighty warrior fighting with you through the pain, and He is there to hold you through every contraction and through every stage of labor, whether it goes according to your birth plan or not. He's been with you throughout your entire pregnancy, and He will continue to be with you as you give birth to and parent your baby. My prayer for you is that as you bring your new little one into the world, you would sense the sacredness of the work you're doing with God and that it would be an experience that takes you deeper into His heart.

A LITTLE PRAYER FOR YOU

Father God, thank You for Your love for me, Your care over me this entire pregnancy, and Your presence with me in all circumstances. Help me experience You more deeply and profoundly in childbirth and to trust Your heart for me and my baby.

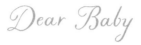

Dear Baby

In your final prebirth letter to your baby, describe what you are thinking and feeling as you prepare to meet your little miracle.

YOUR SPIRITUAL BIRTH PLAN

Our minds, bodies, and spirits are connected in complex ways, and this is especially true in childbirth. Feeling relaxed and loved produces the hormone oxytocin, which is a natural pain reliever, so you may have invited someone you love and trust to help keep you relaxed and breathing during labor. However, while you may have a physical birth plan in place to help your body in labor, do you have a spiritual birth plan to help center your heart on Christ?

Inviting the peace of Christ into your labor room is a powerful way to experience God's presence. You might softly play worship songs, have your birth partner pray over you, or display Bible verses to encourage you. You can prepare a short prayer that you can cry out in your moments of fear or have a battery-powered candle to remind you of His presence with you. Even if you have a planned (or unplanned) cesarean section, consider a strategy for anchoring your hope to God in the operating room.

Strange as it may seem, childbirth can be a worshipful experience. Begin thinking about your spiritual birth plan now, so you can be assured of God's love for you and receive His peace in labor.

PASTE
PHOTO
HERE

BUMP PHOTO

PASTE
PHOTO
HERE

MOM AND BABY'S FIRST PHOTO TOGETHER

LOVE BEYOND
MEASURE

Congratulations! Your baby is finally here! Life has probably been a whirlwind since the birth as you juggle feeding your baby and yourself, sporadic sleep, and welcoming visitors who want to meet your little one. This month, you will be recovering from childbirth, processing your birth story, figuring out new household routines, and trying to manage hormonal fluctuations, all while getting to know this precious tiny person in your arms. As you navigate the early weeks of motherhood, celebrate what has happened, cherish these present moments, and anticipate the joy ahead of you.

WEEK

1

Your beautiful newborn is working hard to figure out life out-side the womb. They need to learn the brand-new new skill of eating for nourishment, whether by breast or bottle, and your baby may constantly need the warmth and safety of your arms. Your breasts will give small amounts of nutrient-rich colostrum at first, then milk may come rushing in after two or three days. Take it very easy this week as your body recovers from birth, and allow yourself plenty of time to just cuddle your baby and soak in the joy of this new tiny wonder.

"A woman giving birth to a child has pain because her time has come; but when her baby is born she forgets the anguish because of her joy that a child is born into the world." John 16:21

JOY ON THE OTHER SIDE

If you're like most women, giving birth was probably one of the most challenging things you've ever done. But the challenges aren't over! As your body recovers, you'll be constantly reminded of all you went through. Perhaps you're wearing very stylish, special underwear from the hospital to cover your sore bottom or trying to nurse a baby while protecting an incision site. Your breasts may be engorged and painful this week, your baby may struggle to take breast or bottle, and your uterus may be cramping as it shrinks back to its normal size. Add sleep deprivation and difficulty sparing time for a shower, and this may not be your most glamorous week! Despite all this, your baby is here, and you have much to celebrate and rejoice over.

As Jesus spent His last hours with His disciples the night of His arrest, He used the comparison of a woman giving birth to help them navigate their emotions. They would grieve when He left them, but He promised to return to them and restore their joy. Jesus added that no one would ever be able to take away the disciples' joy upon His return. In the same way, a woman in labor experiences pain and grief and bewilderment, but all that diminishes when her baby finally arrives.

Even amid the pain and discomfort of labor and your first week postpartum, you likely feel a great deal of delight as you count tiny fingers and toes, gaze at your baby's sweet face as they sleep, and maybe even cry tears of joy as you think of all you've already been through together. What an incredible thing you've done with God: created life, nurtured it with your body, then brought it into the world with great effort and hard work. This week may be filled with physical discomfort, but nothing can take away the joy experienced by a mother holding her newborn.

Perhaps your pregnancy and birth experiences could be likened to a death-and-resurrection scenario, like Jesus' crucifixion. Maybe your pregnancy was difficult, or your labor was excruciating or scary, but the arrival of your baby was like a joyous return from the depths of despair. Perhaps you enjoyed pregnancy and had a great childbirth experience—wonderful! Wherever your experiences have taken you, like Jesus, you have faced great difficulty and emerged victorious. And now what a gift of joy you have to enjoy on the other side.

A LITTLE PRAYER FOR YOU

Lord, thank You for this precious baby! Thank You for bringing me through pregnancy and childbirth, for watching over us both, and for the joy of this new little life. Help my body heal and give me strength for the days ahead.

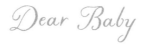

Dear Baby

Write a letter to your baby with your
first thoughts and feelings on meeting them and
about your first moments together.

WEEK
2

In the second week, your baby may hit their first growth spurt and may seem fussier and hungrier. Newborns need up to 17 hours of sleep per day to help them grow, and they may want you to hold them for much of that! Between all the feedings, constant cuddling, and changing diapers, you may wonder where the day goes. Resist any guilt over not doing "enough," whether it's the dishes or reading your Bible. Your prayers may feel jumbled since you're not getting normal sleep. It's okay—this is a brief season, and He is there with you!

And we know that in all things God works for the good of those who love him, who have been called according to his purpose. For those God foreknew he also predestined to be conformed to the image of his Son. Romans 8:28–29

THE AUTHOR OF YOUR BIRTH STORY

Every birth story is different, and you may be contemplating your own as you rock your baby, pace to soothe their cries, or spend hours feeding them. Maybe everything went as you'd planned and dreamed, free of complications and more joyful and beautiful than you'd imagined. Perhaps all your expectations went out the window, decisions felt out of your control, and maybe you're even dealing with trauma. Many women land somewhere in between—with much to remember with both joy and sorrow.

One of the best practices after any major event is processing the story verbally, both with God and with others. What happened? Who was there? How did you feel about it? What happened that you didn't expect? Childbirth is a significant event in your life, a crucial chapter in your story. You might feel the urge to repeat the details over and over with everyone you see, but this is your mind trying to process what happened, so keep telling your story!

In the book of Romans, Paul writes that God, in His sovereignty and providence, manages all things for the good of those who love Him. God is working toward His goal of conforming you with the image of Jesus Christ, making you more and more like Him. When you read this beautiful passage in its context, you find that Paul wasn't talking about God's work just in joyful moments. In fact, God is working for our good *especially* in hardship and suffering. He is the author of your whole story but also the author of your birth story. He was there with you as you gave birth whether it happened as you expected or not. As you process your story and go over the details, ask Him to show you where He was and thank Him for His presence.

Your birth story may be quite emotional—as it should be! Strong emotions are appropriate for such a profound moment in your life. Praise, thanksgiving, worship, lament, grief, anger—all of these are normal and valid emotions and can be brought to Him. As you tell your story, pay attention to what is happening within your heart. Ask for understanding when you need it and read through the Psalms for help in voicing your feelings before God. God is the author of your story, and even if it was difficult, He will use it to shape you into the image of His Son.

A LITTLE PRAYER FOR YOU

Lord, I am grateful that You are the author of my story and that there is never a moment when I am separated from You or outside Your care. Help me process and tell my story and to see where You were working in it.

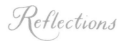

Reflections

Write out the details of your birth story.
How were your expectations met or let down,
and how do you feel about what happened?

WEEK

3

This week, you may notice your baby concentrating on the things around them. Their eyesight is developing rapidly, so they're now able to see the mobile above their crib or the ceiling fan whirring around. After birth, many moms feel a cloud of sadness and loneliness weighing them down as their hormones make radical shifts. Guilt may then flood them for feeling down at such a joyful time! While you may be confused at all that is going on within you, remember that God knows your heart and He wants you to simply bring it to Him, whether it is elated or melancholy.

Why, my soul, are you downcast? Why so disturbed within me? Put your hope in God, for I will yet praise him, my Savior and my God.

Psalm 42:5

BABY BLUES

In the first few weeks postpartum, many women experience what is sometimes called the "baby blues." Between the overwhelming demands of a newborn, the physical exhaustion and struggle for recovery, and the postpartum hormones flooding your body, you may feel a sense of grief and sadness rather than the happiness you thought you'd be experiencing now. There are a lot of changes and challenges as a mother of a newborn! When your baby hits a sudden growth spurt, you may feel trapped underneath a baby who wants to constantly eat. Getting out of the house is a lot of work now, as you have to time naps and feedings correctly and make sure you don't forget anything. You may feel isolated and desperate for adult conversation. Maybe there is a sense of loss over the way things used to be. Maybe you also feel guilty for feeling like this.

David's Psalms are so comforting because they never shy away from the tumultuous emotions every human feels. He asks himself, "Why are you downcast, my soul?" You may be asking yourself the same "Why?" We don't always understand why we're feeling unhappy, and that's okay! Human souls are complex, and to understand our own selves is sometimes a tremendous difficulty. Allow yourself to feel what you're feeling before God, without any kind of mask, then follow the rest of David's advice: "Put your hope in God, for I will yet praise Him." Although David is feeling downcast, he commands his soul to do what he doesn't feel like doing. David both feels his true emotions and urges himself toward praising God even in his despair.

If you're feeling down, make a plan to help yourself feel better and put your hope in God. Go for a walk if you can—exercise will help strengthen your muscles, and the fresh air and movement will help you feel better. As you walk, invite the Lord to help you sort through your emotions. Use feeding times to connect with the Lord in prayer or to meditate on a short passage of Scripture. And, if you need help, don't hesitate to ask—most people want to help but also don't want to intrude! Finally, if your feelings of sadness intensify and last longer than two weeks, you may have postpartum depression. Please reach out to a trusted friend, your doctor, or a mental health professional for help. There is always hope, and one day you will be cheerfully praising the Lord again.

A LITTLE PRAYER FOR YOU

Lord Jesus, thank You that You are with me through every circumstance and through every emotion. Please give my heart peace and steadfastness, and help me hold on to You through these hormonal shifts and life changes. Please give me connections with others and strength to reach out for help when I need it.

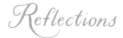

Reflections

Much has changed, and your body, mind,
and soul have been through a lot! Take some time to
journal and pray about how you're feeling.

WEEK
4

Your baby probably gets excited when they see or hear you, and those sweet little smiles should be coming in just a few weeks. They are likely holding their head up a bit and bringing their hands to their mouth, showing significant development in the past few weeks! Many babies are welcomed into the church community, whether through baptism or dedication, depending on your denominational traditions. Ask your church leader about this special rite of passage as you consider the profound task ahead of you as a parent. You need your village of faith to help you, encourage you, and be there for your child.

Start children off on the way they should go, and even when they are old they will not turn from it.

Proverbs 22:6

A GREAT COMMISSION

When God called Abraham to follow Him, His intent was to bless the entire world through Abraham's offspring. Thousands of years later, Jesus was born through Abraham's family. Through Jesus, all people can be reconciled to God in Christ and receive the eternal blessings that come from living as His children. Just before He ascended into heaven, Jesus commissioned His followers to go and make disciples of all nations, baptizing and teaching them in Jesus' ways. He also promised He would be with His people to the very end as they carried out this sacred commission.

As followers of Jesus, we live within this commission to invite others into the presence of God and to enable them to find true eternal blessing in Christ. While we may initially think of foreign missionaries when hearing this Great Commission, these commands are meant for all Jesus' followers, wherever they find themselves.

Your task as a parent is no less spiritual than a missionary's. You are given a great and sacred commission from God to raise this child in His ways, to teach your child to obey Jesus' commands, and to show your child what it means to live in God's presence as His people. As we discussed in week 35 of this devotional, your children will grow up as imitators of your actions and words. What actions are you doing and what words are you using to show your child how to follow God? Demonstrate how

God has blessed you throughout your child's growing-up years, and when your child is grown, you can send them out into the world to bless those they meet, for God's glory.

With this final reflection on your journey through pregnancy and postpartum, I want to bless you as you carry out the holy work ahead of you as a mother:

May God show you the incomparable riches of
His grace through His Son, Jesus Christ.

May your parenting reflect the goodness
of the Father, who created you.

May your baby grow and develop in that same grace, and
may your child always live in the goodness of God.

May the Holy Spirit enable you to lay hold of the
courage He offers you in His presence.

And may God make you and your child a blessing
to the world, to the glory of His name.

A LITTLE PRAYER FOR YOU

Lord, what a sacred commission You have given me as a mother to this child. I pray that You would guide me as I embark on this new adventure. Help me raise this child to love You, to obey You, and to bless the world in Your name.

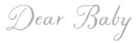

Dear Baby

Write a letter to your baby explaining your
hopes and dreams for your life together, and include
a prayer over your child for their future.

CHRISTIAN LULLABIES

Even if you're not a fabulous singer, lullabies are important for both mothers and their children in the early years. Gentle singing is soothing and also helps forge deep connections between a mother and her children. Your baby loves to hear the sound of your voice, and coupled with the warmth of your body and gentle rocking, you can impart feelings of peace and love to your baby as they drift off to sleep. Some mothers have even found that the songs they sang to their baby in the womb comfort their baby after birth. If there are any songs you often sang while your baby was in your womb, sing them now and see how your baby responds.

Some older lullabies have strange or even nonsensical lyrics—why is a baby rocking in a treetop, then falling? Christian hymns and simple children's songs can be wonderful alternatives. Even your favorite modern praise and worship songs can become lullabies. Here are some suggestions to get you singing:

"Jesus Loves Me"

"Softly and Tenderly Jesus Is Calling"

"How Deep the Father's Love for Us"

"Jesus Paid It All"

"Amazing Grace"

"How Great Thou Art"

"Holy, Holy, Holy"

"On Eagle's Wings"

PASTE
FOOTPRINTS
HERE

BABY'S FOOTPRINTS

ABOUT THE AUTHOR

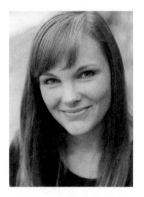

AUBRY G. SMITH, CD AND CBE (CBI), is a certified childbirth educator and birth doula who received her master's in theological studies at Columbia International University. Passionate about the intersection of Biblical theology, spiritual formation, and the profound experience of childbirth, she is also the author of *Holy Labor: How Childbirth Shapes a Woman's Soul.* Aubry also works for an international Christian nonprofit organization. Having spent five years in the Middle East training cross-cultural workers and offering birth services to expats, she and her husband now provide support services for refugees resettled in the United Kingdom. Aubry lives with her husband and three children in Belfast, Northern Ireland. Visit her online at aubrygsmith.com.